ABC OF CLINICAL HAEMATOLOGY

ABC OF CLINICAL HAEMATOLOGY

Edited by

DREW PROVAN

Consultant Haematologist and Honorary Senior Lecturer
Southampton University Hospitals NHS Trust, Southampton
and

ANDREW HENSON

General Practitioner, Southampton

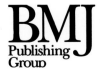

BMJ
Publishing
Group

© BMJ Publishing Group 1998

First published in 1998
Reprinted 1999
by the BMJ Publishing Group, BMA House, Tavistock Square,
London WC1H 9JR

British Library Cataloguing in Publication Data

A catalogue record for this book is available from the British Library

ISBN 0 7279 1206 2

Typeset by Apek Typesetters Ltd., Nailsea, Bristol
Printed and bound by Craft Print, Singapore

Contents

Page

Contributors vii
Preface ix

 1 **Iron deficiency anaemia**   1
   Rebecca Frewin, Andrew Henson, *and* Drew Provan
 2 **Macrocytic anaemias**   5
   Victor Hoffbrand, *and* Drew Provan
 3 **The hereditary anaemias** 10
   David J Weatherall
 4 **Polycythaemia, primary (essential) thrombocythaemia**
   and myelofibrosis 16
   Maria Messinezy, *and* TC Pearson
 5 **Chronic myeloid leukaemia** 20
   John Goldman
 6 **The acute leukaemias** 24
   RJ Liesner, *and* AH Goldstone
 7 **Platelet disorders** 29
   RJ Liesner, *and* SJ Machin
 8 **The myelodysplastic syndromes** 34
   David G Oscier
 9 **Multiple myeloma and related conditions** 39
   Charles RJ Singer
10 **Bleeding disorders, thrombosis, and anticoagulation** . . 43
   KK Hampton, *and* FE Preston
11 **Malignant lymphomas and chronic lymphocytic**
   leukaemia 47
   GM Mead
12 **Bone marrow and stem cell transplantation** 51
   Andrew Duncombe
13 **Haematological disorders at the extremes of life** 56
   Adrian C Newland, *and* Tyrrell GJR Evans
14 **Haematological emergencies** 60
   Rebecca Frewin, Andrew Henson, *and* Drew Provan
15 **The future of haematology, molecular biology, and gene** 65
   therapy . . . .
   Adele K Fielding, Sally Ager, *and* Stephen J Russell
   Index 71

CONTRIBUTORS

Sally Ager
Kay Kendall Leukaemia Fund Clinical Research Fellow
Department of Haematology, University of Cambridge, MRC Centre, Cambridge

Andrew Duncombe
Consultant Haematologist
Southampton University Hospitals NHS Trust, Southampton

Tyrrell G J R Evans
Senior Lecturer
Department of General Practice and Primary Care, King's College School of Medicine
and Dentistry, London

Adele K Fielding
Leukaemia Research Fund Clinical Research Fellow
Department of Haematology, University of Cambridge, MRC Centre, Cambridge

Rebecca Frewin
Supernumerary Specialist Registrar in Haematology
Musgrove Park Hospital, Taunton, Somerset

John Goldman
Professor of Haematology
Imperial College School of Medicine, Hammersmith Hospital, London

A H Goldstone
Consultant Haematologist
Department of Haematology, University College London Hospitals NHS Trust, London

K K Hampton
Senior Lecturer in Haematology
Royal Hallamshire Hospital, Sheffield

Andrew Henson
General Practitioner
Southampton

Victor Hoffbrand
Emeritus Professor of Haematology and Honorary Consultant Haematologist
Royal Free Hospital Hampstead NHS Trust and School of Medicine, London

R J Liesner
Senior Registrar
Department of Haematology and Oncology, Great Ormond Street, Hospital for Children
NHS Trust, London

S J Machin
Professor of Haematology
University College London Hospitals NHS Trust, London

G M Mead
Consultant in Medical Oncology
Wessex Medical Oncology Unit, Royal South Hants Hospital, Southampton

Maria Messinezy
Clinical Assistant in Haematology
United Medical and Dental Schools of Guy's and Thomas's Hospitals, London

Adrian C Newland
Professor of Haematology
St Bartholomew's and the Royal London School of Medicine and Dentistry, London

David G Oscier
Consultant Haematologist
Department of Haematology and Oncology, Royal Bournemouth Hospital,
Bournemouth, and Honorary Senior Lecturer, University of Southampton

T C Pearson
Professor of Haematology
United Medical and Dental Schools of Guy's and St Thomas's Hospitals, London

F E Preston
Professor of Haematology
Royal Hallamshire Hospital, Sheffield

Drew Provan
Consultant Haematologist and Honorary Senior Lecturer
Southampton University Hospitals NHS Trust, Southampton

Stephen J Russell
MRC Senior Scientist and Honorary Consultant
Department of Haematology, University of Cambridge, MRC Centre, Cambridge

Charles R J Singer
Consultant Haematologist
Royal United Hospital, Bath

Sir David J Weatherall
Regius Professor of Medicine
Institute of Molecular Medicine, University of Oxford, John Radcliffe Hospital, Oxford

Preface

Clinical haematology is a fast moving and exciting specialty embracing aspects of pathology, general medicine, cancer and molecular science. We aim with this book to provide an overview of the subject highlighting recent advances, and have been fortunate in obtaining up to date, succinct contributions from leading haematologists in the UK.

This book is intended to cover the areas most relevant to non-specialists, for example, junior hospital doctors, and general practitioners responsible for the care of patients with blood related problems. It will also be of value to doctors studying for the MRCP diploma, haematology trainees, nurses on medical or haematology units, and technical staff within haematology or blood transfusion laboratories.

We enjoyed writing and editing this book immensely, and extend warm thanks to the many distinguished colleagues who made it possible. It is hoped the enthusiasm of the contributors will be evident and perhaps stimulate the reader to explore clinical haematology in greater detail.

Drew Provan and Andrew Henson

1 IRON DEFICIENCY ANAEMIA

Rebecca Frewin, Andrew Henson, Drew Provan

> Diagnosing iron deficiency is usually straightforward—the major challenge is determining the cause of the anaemia

Iron deficiency is the commonest cause of anaemia worldwide and is frequently seen in general practice. The anaemia of iron deficiency is caused by defective synthesis of haemoglobin, resulting in red cells that are smaller than normal (microcytic) and contain reduced amounts of haemoglobin (hypochromic).

Iron metabolism

Daily dietary iron requirements per 24 hours

Male	1 mg
Adolescence	2-3 mg
Female (reproductive age)	2-3 mg
Pregnancy	3-4 mg
Infancy	1 mg
Maximum bioavailability from normal diet about	4 mg

Iron has a pivotal role in many metabolic processes, and the average adult contains 3-5 g of iron, of which two thirds is in the oxygen-carrying molecule haemoglobin.

A normal Western diet provides about 15 mg of iron daily, of which 5-10% is absorbed, principally in the duodenum and upper jejunum, where the acidic conditions help the absorption of iron in the ferrous form. Absorption is helped by the presence of other reducing substances, such as hydrochloric acid and ascorbic acid. The body has the capacity to increase its iron absorption in the face of increased demand—for example, in pregnancy, lactation, growth spurts, and iron deficiency.

Once absorbed from the bowel, iron is transported across the mucosal cell to the blood, where it is carried by the protein transferrin to developing red cells in the bone marrow. Iron stores comprise ferritin, a labile and readily accessible source of iron, and haemosiderin, an insoluble form found predominantly in macrophages.

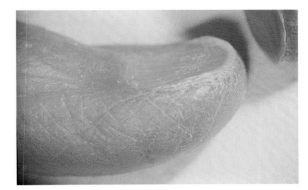

Figure 1.1 Nail changes in iron deficiency anaemia (koilonychia).

About 1 mg of iron a day is shed from the body in urine, faeces, sweat, and cells shed from the skin and gastrointestinal tract. Menstrual losses of an additional 20 mg a month and the increased requirements of pregnancy (500-1000 mg) contribute to the higher incidence of iron deficiency in women of reproductive age.

Clinical features of iron deficiency

Risk factors in development of iron deficiency

Age—Infants (especially if history of prematurity); adolescents; postmenopausal women; old age
Sex—Increased risk in women
Reproduction—Menorrhagia
Renal—Haematuria (rarer cause)
Gastrointestinal tract—Appetite or weight changes; changes in bowel habit; bleeding from rectum/melaena; gastric or bowel surgery
Drug history—Especially aspirin and non-steroidal anti-inflammatories
Social history—Diet, especially vegetarians
Physiological—Pregnancy; infancy; adolescence; breast feeding; age of weaning

The symptoms accompanying iron deficiency depend on how rapidly the anaemia develops. In cases of chronic, slow blood loss, the body adapts to the increasing anaemia, and patients can often tolerate extremely low concentrations of haemoglobin—for example, < 70 g/l — with remarkably few symptoms. Most patients complain of increasing lethargy and dyspnoea. More unusual symptoms are headaches, tinnitus, and taste disturbance.

On examination, several skin, nail, and other epithelial changes may be seen in chronic iron deficiency. Atrophy of the skin occurs in about a third of patients, and nail changes such as koilonychia (spoon shaped nails) result in brittle, flattened nails. Patients may also complain of angular stomatitis, in which painful cracks appear at the angle of the mouth, sometimes accompanied by glossitis. Although uncommon,

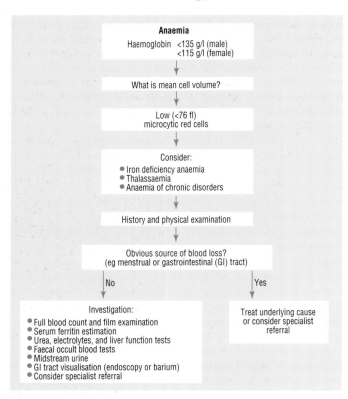

Figure 1.2 Diagnosis and investigation of iron deficiency anaemia.

The flowchart reads:

Anaemia
Haemoglobin <135 g/l (male)
<115 g/l (female)

↓

What is mean cell volume?

↓

Low (<76 fl)
microcytic red cells

↓

Consider:
● Iron deficiency anaemia
● Thalassaemia
● Anaemia of chronic disorders

↓

History and physical examination

↓

Obvious source of blood loss?
(eg menstrual or gastrointestinal (GI) tract)

No ↓   Yes ↓

Investigation:
● Full blood count and film examination
● Serum ferritin estimation
● Urea, electrolytes, and liver function tests
● Faecal occult blood tests
● Midstream urine
● GI tract visualisation (endoscopy or barium)
● Consider specialist referral

Treat underlying cause or consider specialist referral

Causes of iron deficiency anaemia

Reproductive system
● Menorrhagia

Gastrointestinal tract
Bleeding
● Oesophagitis
● Oesophageal varices
● Hiatus hernia
● Peptic ulcer
● Inflammatory bowel disease
● Haemorrhoids
● Carcinoma: stomach, colorectal
● Angiodysplasia
● hereditary haemorrhagic telangiectasia (rare)

Malabsorption
● Coeliac disease
● Atrophic gastritis (also may result *from* iron deficiency)

Physiological
● Growth spurts (especially in premature infants)
● Pregnancy

Dietary
● Vegans
● Elderly

Genitourinary system
● Haematuria (?cause)

Worldwide commonest cause of iron deficiency is hookworm infection

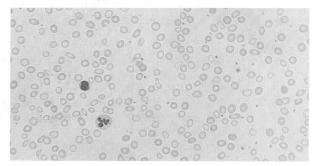

Figure 1.3 Blood film showing changes of iron deficiency anaemia.

oesophageal and pharyngeal webs can be a feature of iron deficiency anaemia (consider this in middle aged women presenting with dysphagia). These changes are believed to be due to a reduction in the iron-containing enzymes in the epithelium and gastrointestinal tract.

Tachycardia and cardiac failure may occur with severe anaemia, and in such cases prompt remedial action should be taken.

When iron deficiency is confirmed a full clinical history including leading questions on possible gastrointestinal blood loss or malabsorption (as in, for example, coeliac disease) should be obtained. Menstrual losses should be assessed, and the importance of dietary factors and regular blood donation should not be overlooked.

Diet alone is seldom the sole cause for iron deficiency anaemia in Britain except when it prevents an adequate response to a physiological challenge—as in pregnancy, for example.

Laboratory investigations

Differential diagnosis of hypochromic anaemia

Factor	Iron deficiency	Chronic disorders	Thalassaemia trait (α or β)	Sideroblastic anaemia
Degree of anaemia	Any	Seldom <90 g/l	Mild	Any
Mean cell volume	↓	N or ↓	↓↓	N, ↓ or ↑
Serum ferritin	↓	N or ↑	N	↑
TIBC	↑	↓	N	N
Serum iron	↓	↓	N	↑
Marrow iron	Absent	Present	Present	Present

N = normal; TIBC = total iron binding capacity

A full blood count and film should be taken. These will confirm the anaemia; recognising the indices of iron deficiency is usually straightforward (reduced haemoglobin concentration, reduced mean cell volume, reduced mean cell haemoglobin, reduced mean cell haemoglobin concentration). The blood film shows microcytic hypochromic red cells. Hypochromic anaemia occurs in other disorders, such as anaemia of chronic disorders and sideroblastic anaemias and in globin synthesis disorders, such as thalassaemia. To help to differentiate the type, further haematinic assays may be necessary. Difficulties in

Investigations in iron deficiency anaemia

- Full clinical history and physical examination
- Full blood count and blood film examination
- Haematinic assays (serum ferritin, vitamin B_{12}, folate)
- Urea and electrolytes, liver function tests
- Faecal occult bloods
- Midstream urine (occult blood loss)
- Fibreoptic and/or barium studies of gastrointestinal tract
- Pelvic ultrasound (females, if indicated)

Diagnosis of iron deficiency anaemia

Reduced haemoglobin	Men <135 g/l, women <115 g/l
Reduced mean cell volume	<76 fl
Reduced mean cell haemoglobin	29·5 ± 2·5 pg
Reduced mean cell haemoglobin concentration	325 ± 25 g/l
Blood film	Microcytic hypochromic red cells with pencil cells and target cells
Reduced serum ferritin*	Men <10 µg/l, women (postmenopausal) <10 µg/l, (premenopausal) <5 µg/l
Reduced serum iron*	Men <14 µmol/l, women <11 µmol/l
Increased serum iron and total binding capacity*	>75 µmol/l

*Check with local laboratory for reference ranges

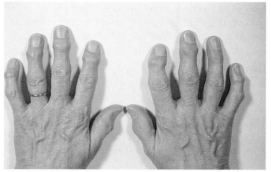

Figure 1.4 Patient with osteoarthritis (Heberden's nodes). This patient was iron deficient. Her non-steroidal anti-inflammatory drugs had caused gastrointestinal bleeding.

diagnosis arise when more than one type of anaemia is present—for example, iron deficiency and folate deficiency in malabsorption, in a population where thalassaemia is present, or in pregnancy, when the interpretation of red cell indices may be difficult.

Haematinic assays will demonstrate reduced serum ferritin concentration in straightforward iron deficiency. As an acute phase protein, however, the serum ferritin concentration may be normal or even raised in inflammatory or malignant disease.

A prime example of this is found in rheumatoid disease, in which active disease may result in a spuriously raised serum ferritin concentration masking an underlying iron deficiency caused by gastrointestinal bleeding after non-steroidal analgesic treatment. There may also be confusion in liver disease as the liver contains stores of ferritin that are released after hepatocellular damage, leading to raised serum ferritin concentrations. In cases where ferritin estimation is likely to be misleading, it can be helpful to determine the serum iron concentration and total iron binding capacity, which are reduced and raised respectively in uncomplicated iron deficiency. In common with serum ferritin estimation, however, these measures are often difficult to interpret when inflammation is present.

Diagnostic bone marrow sampling is seldom performed in simple iron deficiency, but if the diagnosis is in doubt a marrow aspirate may be carried out to demonstrate absent bone marrow stores.

When iron deficiency has been diagnosed, the underlying cause should be investigated and treated. Often the history will indicate the likely source of bleeding—for example, menstrual blood loss or gastrointestinal bleeding. If there is no obvious cause, further investigation generally depends on the age and sex of the patient. In male patients and postmenopausal women possible gastrointestinal blood loss is investigated by performing faecal occult bloods and visualisation of the gastrointestinal tract (endoscopic or barium studies). Faecal occult bloods are useful screening tests (sensitivity 50-75% in the detection of colorectal cancer), but a negative result should not preclude other investigations of the gastrointestinal tract.

Management

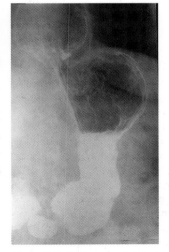

Figure 1.5 Barium meal showing hiatus hernia leading to iron deficiency anaemia.

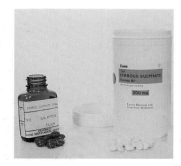

Figure 1.6 Oral iron replacement therapy.

Effective management of iron deficiency relies on (A) the appropriate management of the underlying cause (for example, gastro-intestinal or menstrual blood loss) and (B) iron replacement therapy.

Oral iron replacement therapy with gradual replenishment of iron stores and restoration of haemoglobin is the preferred treatment. Oral ferrous salts are the treatment of choice (ferric salts are less well absorbed) and usually takes the form of ferrous sulphate 200 mg three times daily (providing 65 mg×3 = 195 mg elemental iron/day). Alternative preparations include ferrous gluconate and ferrous fumarate. All three compounds, however, are associated with a high incidence of side effects, including nausea, constipation, and diarrhoea. These side effects may be reduced by taking the tablets after meals, but even milder symptoms account for poor compliance with oral iron supplementation. Modified release preparations have been developed to reduce side effects but in practice prove expensive and often release the iron beyond the sites of optimal absorption.

Effective iron replacement therapy should result in a rise in haemoglobin concentration of around 1 g/l per day (about 20 g/l every three weeks), but this varies from patient to patient. Once the haemoglobin concentration is within the normal range, iron replacement should continue for three months to replenish the iron stores.

Failure to respond to oral iron therapy

Elemental iron content of various oral iron preparations

Preparation	Amount (mg)	Ferrous iron (mg)
Ferrous fumarate	200	65
Ferrous gluconate	300	35
Ferrous succinate	100	35
Ferrous sulphate	300	60
Ferrous sulphate (dried)	200	65

Intravenous iron preparations

- Intravenous iron preparations are available in Britain on a named patient basis only
- These preparations are frequently associated with side effects, some of which are severe—such as anaphylaxis
- They should therefore be given only under close medical supervision and when full resuscitation facilities are available

The rise in haemoglobin concentration is no faster with parenteral iron preparations than with oral iron therapy

Drs A G Smith and A Amos provided the photographic material and Dr A Odurny provided the radiograph. The source of the detail in the table is the *British National Formulary*, No 32(Sep), 1995.

The main reason for failure to respond to oral iron therapy is poor compliance. However, if the losses (for example, bleeding) exceed the amount of iron absorbed daily, the haemoglobin concentration will not rise as expected; this will also be the case in combined deficiency states.

The presence of underlying inflammation or malignancy may also lead to a poor response to therapy. Finally, an incorrect diagnosis of iron deficiency anaemia should be considered in patients who fail to respond adequately to iron replacement therapy.

Intravenous and intramuscular iron preparations

Parenteral iron may be used when the patient cannot tolerate oral supplements—for example, when patients have severe gastrointestinal side effects or if the losses exceed the daily amount that can be absorbed orally.

Iron sorbitol injection is a complex of iron, sorbitol and citric acid. Treatment consists of a course of deep intramuscular injections. The dosage varies from patient to patient and depends on (A) the initial haemoglobin concentration and (B) body weight. Generally, 10-20 deep intramuscular injections are given over two to three weeks. Apart from being painful, the injections also lead to skin staining at the site of injection and arthralgia.

Alternative treatments

Blood transfusion is not indicated unless the patient has decompensated due to a drop in haemoglobin concentration and needs a more rapid rise in haemoglobin—for example, in cases of worsening angina or severe coexisting pulmonary disease. In cases of iron deficiency with serious ongoing acute bleeding, blood transfusion may be required.

Prevention

When absorption from the diet is likely to be matched or exceeded by losses, extra sources of iron should be considered—for example, prophylactic iron supplements in pregnancy or after gastrectomy or encouragement of breast feeding or use of formula milk during the first year of life (rather than cows' milk, which is a poor source of iron).

2 MACROCYTIC ANAEMIAS

Victor Hoffbrand, Drew Provan

Macrocytosis is a rise in the mean cell volume of the red cells above the normal range (in adults 80-95 fl (femtolitres)). It is detected with a blood count, in which the mean cell volume, as well as other red cell indices, is measured. The mean cell volume is lower in children than in adults, with a normal mean of 70 fl at age 1 year, rising by about 1 fl each year until adult volumes are reached at puberty.

The causes of macrocytosis fall into two groups: (a) deficiency of vitamin B_{12} (cobalamin) or folate (or rarely abnormalities of their metabolism) in which the bone marrow is megaloblastic and (b) other causes, in which the bone marrow is usually normoblastic. In this article the two groups are considered separately, and then the reader is taken through the steps to diagnose the cause of macrocytosis and its management.

> Megaloblastic bone marrow is exemplified by developing red blood cells that are larger than normal, with nuclei more immature than their cytoplasm. The underlying mechanism is defective DNA synthesis

Deficiency of vitamin B_{12} or folate

Causes of megaloblastic anaemia

Diet
Vitamin B_{12} deficiency—Veganism, poor quality diet
Folate deficiency—Poor quality diet, old age, poverty, synthetic diet without added folic acid, goats' milk

Malabsorption
Gastric causes of vitamin B_{12} deficiency—Pernicious anaemia, congenital intrinsic factor deficiency, gastrectomy
Intestinal causes of vitamin B_{12} deficiency—Stagnant loop, congenital selective malabsorption, ileal resection, Crohn's disease
Intestinal causes of folate deficiency—gluten induced enteropathy, tropical sprue, jejunal resection

Increased cell turnover
Folate deficiency—Pregnancy, prematurity, chronic haemolytic anaemia (such as sickle cell anaemia), extensive inflammatory and malignant diseases

Renal loss
Folate deficiency—Congestive cardiac failure, dialysis

Drugs
Folate deficiency—Anticonvulsants, sulphasalazine

Defects of vitamin B_{12} metabolism—for example, transcobalamin II deficiency, nitrous oxide anaesthesia-or of folate metabolism (such as methotrexate treatment), or rare inherited defects of DNA synthesis may all cause megaloblastic anaemia

Other causes of macrocytosis*

- Alcohol
- Liver disease
- Hypothyroidism
- Reticulocytosis
- Aplastic anaemia
- Red cell aplasia
- Myelodysplasia
- Cytotoxic drugs
- Paraproteinaemia (such as myeloma)
- Pregnancy
- Neonatal period

* These are usually associated with a normoblastic marrow

Vitamin B_{12} deficiency

The body's requirement for vitamin B_{12} is about 1 µg daily. This is amply supplied by a normal Western diet (vitamin B_{12} content 10-30 µg daily) but not by a strict vegan diet, which excludes all animal produce (including milk, eggs, and cheese). Absorption of vitamin B_{12} is through the ileum, facilitated by intrinsic factor, which is secreted by the parietal cells of the stomach. Absorption is limited to 2-3 µg daily.

In Britain, vitamin B_{12} deficiency is usually due to pernicious anaemia, which now accounts for up to 80% of all cases of megaloblastic anaemia. The incidence of the disease is 1:10 000 in northern Europe, and the disease occurs in all races. The underlying mechanism is an autoimmune gastritis that results in achlorhydria and the absence of intrinsic factor. The incidence of pernicious anaemia peaks at age 60; the condition has a female:male incidence of 1.6:1.0 and is more common in those with early greying, blue eyes, and blood group A, and in those with a family history of the disease or of diseases that may be associated with it—for example, vitiligo, myxoedema, Hashimoto's disease, Addison's disease of adrenal, and hypoparathyroidism.

Other causes of vitamin B_{12} deficiency are infrequent in Britain. Veganism is an unusual cause of severe deficiency as most vegetarians and vegans include some vitamin B_{12} in their diet. Moreover, unlike in pernicious anaemia, the enterohepatic circulation for vitamin B_{12} is intact in vegans, so vitamin B_{12} stores are conserved. Gastric resection and intestinal causes of malabsorption of vitamin B_{12}—for example, ileal resection or the intestinal stagnant loop syndrome—are less common

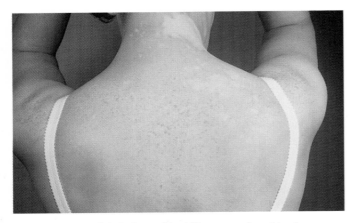

Figure 2.1 Patient with vitiligo on neck and back.

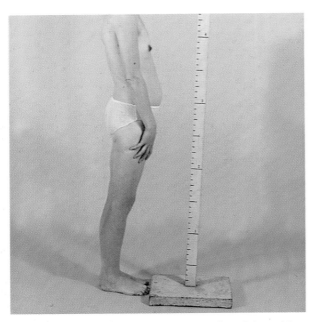

Figure 2.2 Patient with coeliac disease: underweight and low stature.

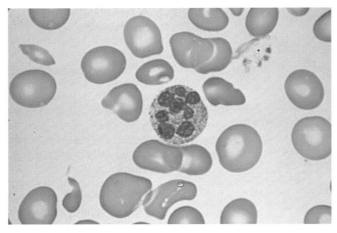

Figure 2.3 Blood film in vitamin B$_{12}$ deficiency showing macrocytic red cells and a hypersegmented neutrophil.

now that abdominal tuberculosis is infrequent and H2-antagonists have been introduced for treating peptic ulceration, thus reducing the need for gastrectomy.

Folate deficiency

The daily requirement for folate is 100-200 µg, and a normal mixed diet contains about 200-300 µg. Natural folates are largely in the polyglutamate form, and these are absorbed through the upper small intestine after deconjugation and conversion to the monoglutamate 5-methyl tetrahydrofolate.

Body stores are sufficient for only about four months. Folate deficiency may arise because of inadequate dietary intake, malabsorption (especially gluten induced enteropathy), or excessive use as proliferating cells degrade folate. Deficiency in pregnancy may be due partly to inadequate diet, partly to transfer of folate to the fetus, and partly to increased folate degradation.

Consequences of vitamin B$_{12}$ or folate deficiencies

Megaloblastic anaemia—Clinical features include pallor and jaundice. The onset is gradual, and a severely anaemic patient may present in congestive heart failure or only when an infection supervenes. The blood film shows oval macrocytes and hypersegmented neutrophil nuclei (with six lobes). In severe cases, the white cell count and platelet count also fall (pancytopenia). The bone marrow shows characteristic megaloblastic erythroblasts and giant metamyelocytes (early granulocyte precursors). Biochemically, there is an increase in plasma of unconjugated bilirubin and serum lactic dehydrogenase, with, in severe cases, an absence of haptoglobins and presence in urine of haemosiderin. These changes, including jaundice, are due to increased destruction of red cell precursors in the marrow (ineffective erythropoiesis).

Vitamin B$_{12}$ neuropathy—A minority of patients with vitamin B$_{12}$ deficiency develop a neuropathy due to symmetrical damage to the peripheral nerves and posterior and lateral columns of the spinal cord, the legs being more affected than the arms. Psychiatric abnormalities and visual disturbance may also occur. Men are more commonly affected than women. The neuropathy may occur in the absence of anaemia. Psychiatric changes and at most a mild peripheral neuropathy may be ascribed to folate deficiency.

Neural tube defects—Folic acid supplements in pregnancy have been shown to reduce the incidence of neural tube defects (spina bifida, encephalocoele and anencephaly) in the fetus and may also reduce the incidence of cleft palate and hare lip. No clear relation exists between the incidence of these defects and folate deficiency in the mother, although the

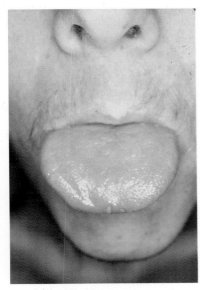

lower the maternal red cell folate (and serum vitamin B_{12}) concentrations even within the normal range, the more likely neural tube defects are to occur in the fetus. One underlying mechanism seems to be a genetic defect in folate metabolism, for example, of 5, 10 methylene tetrahydrofolate reductase.

Gonadal dysfunction—Deficiency of either vitamin B_{12} or folate may cause sterility, which is reversible with appropriate vitamin supplementation.

Epithelial cell changes—Glossitis and other epithelial surfaces may show cytological abnormalities.

Cardiovascular disease—Raised serum homocysteine concentrations have been associated with arterial obstruction and venous thrombosis. An association between low serum folate levels and myocardial infarct has been reported.

Figure 2.4 Glossitis due to vitamin B_{12} deficiency.

Other causes of macrocytosis

Investigations which may be needed in patients with macrocytosis

- Serum B_{12} assay
- Serum and red cell folate assays
- Liver and thyroid function
- Reticulocyte count
- Serum protein electrophoresis
- For vitamin B_{12} deficiency: serum parietal cell and intrinsic factor antibodies, radioactive vitamin B_{12} absorption with and without intrinsic factor (Schilling test), possibly serum gastrin concentration
- For folate defiency: antigliadin, antiendomysial and antireticulin antibodies
- Consider bone marrow examination for megaloblastic changes suggestive of vitamin B_{12} or folate deficiency, or alternative diagnoses—for example, myelodysplasia, aplastic anaemia, myeloma
- Endoscopy—gastric biopsy (vitamin B_{12} deficiency), duodenal biopsy (folate deficiency)

The most common cause of macrocytosis in Britain is alcohol. Fairly small quantities of alcohol—for example, two gin and tonics or half a bottle of wine a day—especially in women, may cause a rise of mean cell volume to > 100 fl, typically without anaemia or any detectable change in liver function.

The mechanism for the rise in mean cell volume is uncertain. In liver disease the volume may rise due to excessive lipid deposition on red cell membranes, and the rise is particularly pronounced in liver disease caused by alcohol. A modest rise in mean cell volume is found in severe thyroid deficiency.

In other causes of macrocytosis, other haematological abnormalities are usually present—in myelodysplasia (a frequent cause of macrocytosis in elderly people) there are usually quantitative or qualitative changes in the white cells and platelets in the blood. In aplastic anaemia, pancytopenia is present; pure red cell aplasia may also cause macrocytosis. Changes in plasma proteins—presence of a paraprotein (as in myeloma)—may cause a rise in mean cell volume without macrocytes being present in the blood film. Physiological causes of macrocytosis are pregnancy and the neonatal period. Drugs that affect DNA synthesis—for example, hydroxyurea and azathioprine—can cause macrocytosis with or without megaloblastic changes. Finally, a rare, benign familial type of macrocytosis has been described.

Diagnosis

Results of absorption tests of radioactive vitamin B_{12}

	Dose of vitamin B_{12} given alone	Dose of vitamin B_{12} given with intrinsic factor
Vegan	Normal	Normal
Pernicious anaemia or gastrectomy	Low	Normal
Ileal resection	Low	Low
Intestinal blind-loop syndrome	Low*	Low*

* Corrected by antibiotics.

Biochemical assays

The most widely used screening tests for the deficiencies are the serum B_{12} and folate assays. A low serum concentration implies a deficiency, but a subnormal serum concentration may occur in the absence of pronounced body deficiency—for example, in pregnancy (vitamin B_{12}) and with very recent poor dietary intake (folate).

Red cell folate can also be used to screen for folate deficiency; a low concentration usually implies appreciable depletion of body folate,

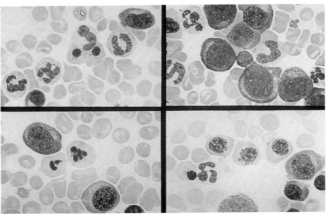

Figure 2.5 Bone marrow appearances in megaloblastic anaemia: developing red cells are larger than normal, with nuclei that are immature relative to their cytoplasm (nuclear:cytoplasmic asynchrony).

but the concentration also falls in severe vitamin B_{12} deficiency, so it is more difficult to interpret the significance of a low red cell than serum folate concentration in patients with megaloblastic anaemia. Moreover, if the patient has received a recent blood transfusion the red cell folate concentration will partly reflect the folate concentration of the transfused red cells.

Specialist investigations

Assays of serum homocysteine (raised in vitamin B_{12} or folate deficiency) or methylmalonic acid (raised in vitamin B_{12} deficiency) are used in some specialised laboratories.

Autoantibodies

For patients with vitamin B_{12} or folate deficiency it is important to establish the underlying cause. In pernicious anaemia, intrinsic factor antibodies are present in plasma in 50% and parietal cell antibodies in 90% of patients. Antigliadin, anti-endomysial and antireticulin antibodies are usually positive in gluten induced enteropathy.

Other investigations

Radioactive vitamin B_{12} absorption studies—for example, Schilling test—show impaired absorption of the vitamin in pernicious anaemia; this can be corrected by giving intrinsic factor. In patients with an intestinal lesion, however, absorption of vitamin B_{12} cannot be corrected with intrinsic factor.

Endoscopy should be performed to confirm atrophic gastritis and exclude gastric carcinoma or gastric polyps, which are two to three times more common in patients with pernicious anaemia than in age and sex matched controls.

A bone marrow examination is usually performed to confirm megaloblastic anaemia. It is also required for the diagnosis of myelodysplasia, aplastic anaemia, myeloma, or other marrow disorders associated with macrocytosis.

If folate deficiency is diagnosed it is important to assess dietary folate intake and to exclude gluten induced enteropathy by endoscopy and duodenal biopsy. The deficiency is common in patients with diseases of increased cell turnover who also have a poor diet.

Treatment

Preventing folate deficiency in pregnancy

- As prophylaxis against folate deficiency in pregnancy, daily doses of folic acid 400 µg are usual
- Larger doses are not recommended as they could mask megaloblastic anaemia due to vitamin B_{12} deficiency and thus allow B_{12} neuropathy to develop
- As neural tube defects occur by the 28th day of pregnancy, it is advisable for a woman's daily folate intake to be increased by 400 µg/day at the time of conception
- Whether this can be achieved by increased consumption of foods with a high folate content—for example, liver, green vegetables, and cereals—or whether women have to take additional folic acid or eat foods deliberately fortified with added folate is the subject of current discussion
- The US Food and Drugs Administration announced in 1996 that specified grain products (including most enriched breads, flours, cornmeal, rice, noodles, and macaroni) will be required to be fortified with folic acid to levels ranging from 0.43 mg to 1.5 mg per pound (453 g) of product
- For mothers who have already had an infant with a neural tube defect, larger doses of folic acid—for example, 5 mg daily—are recommended before and during subsequent pregnancy

Vitamin B_{12} deficiency is treated initially by giving the patient six injections of hydroxocobalamin 1 mg at intervals of about three to four days, followed by four such injections a year for life. For patients undergoing total gastrectomy or ileal resection it is sensible to start the maintenance injections from the time of operation. For vegans, less frequent injections—for example, one or two a year—may be sufficient, and the patient should be advised to eat foods to which vitamin B_{12} has been added, such as certain fortified breads or other foods.

Folate deficiency is treated with folic acid, usually 5 mg daily orally for four months, which is continued only if the underlying cause cannot be corrected. As prophylaxis against folate deficiency in patients with a severe haemolytic anaemia—such as sickle cell anaemia—5 mg folic acid once weekly is probably sufficient. Vitamin B_{12} deficiency must be excluded in all patients starting folic acid treatment at these doses as such treatment may correct the anaemia in vitamin B_{12} deficiency but allow neurological disease to develop.

The illustration of the bone marrow is reproduced with permission from Clinical Haematology (AV Hoffbrand, J Pettit), 2nd ed, London: Mosby International, 1994.

3 THE HEREDITARY ANAEMIAS

David J Weatherall

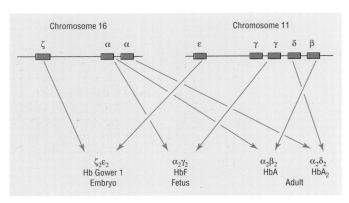

Figure 3.1 Simplified representation of the genetic control of human haemoglobin. Because α chains are shared by both fetal and adult haemoglobin, mutations of the α globin genes affect haemoglobin production in both fetal and adult life; diseases that are due to defective β globin production are only manifest after birth when Hb A replaces Hb F.

Hereditary anaemias include disorders of the structure or synthesis of haemoglobin; deficiencies of enzymes that provide the red cell with energy or protect it from chemical damage; and abnormalities of the proteins of the red cell's membrane. Inherited diseases of haemoglobin, haemoglobinopathies, are by far the most important.

The structure of human haemoglobin (Hb) changes during development. By the 12th week embryonic haemoglobin is replaced by fetal haemoglobin (Hb F), which is slowly replaced after birth by the adult haemoglobins, Hb A and Hb A_2. Each type of haemoglobin consists of two different pairs of peptide chains; Hb A has the structure $\alpha_2\beta_2$ (namely, two α chains plus two β chains), Hb A_2 has the structure of $\alpha_2\delta_2$, and Hb F, $\alpha_2\gamma_2$.

The haemoglobinopathies consist of structural haemoglobin variants (the most important of which are the sickling disorders) and thalassaemias (hereditary defects of the synthesis of either the α or β globin chains).

The sickling disorders

Sickling syndromes

- Hb SS (sickle cell anaemia)
- Hb SC disease
- Hb S/β$^+$ thalassaemia
- Hb S/β° thalassaemia
- Hb SD disease

Sickle cell trait (Hb A and Hb S)

- Less than half the Hb in each red cell is Hb S
- Occasional renal papillary necrosis
- Inability to concentrate the urine (older individuals)
- Red cells do not sickle unless oxygen saturations < 40% (rarely reached in venous blood)
- Painful crises and splenic infraction have been reported in severe hypoxia—such as unpressurised aircraft, anaesthesia

Sickling is more severe where Hb S is present with another β globin chain abnormality—such as Hb S and Hb C (Hb SC) or Hb S and Hb D (Hb SD)

Classification and inheritance

The common sickling disorders consist of the homozygous state for the sickle cell gene—that is, sickle cell anaemia (Hb SS)—and the compound heterozygous state for the sickle cell gene and that for either Hb C (another β chain variant) or β thalassaemia (termed Hb SC disease or sickle cell β thalassaemia). The sickle cell mutation results in a single amino acid substitution in the β globin chain; heterozygotes have one normal (β^A) and one affected β chain (β^S) gene and produce about 60% Hb A and 40% Hb S; homozygotes produce mainly Hb S with small amounts of Hb F. Compound heterozygotes for Hb S and Hb C produce almost equal amounts of each variant, whereas those who inherit the sickle cell gene from one parent and β thalassaemia from the other make predominantly sickle haemoglobin.

Pathophysiology

The amino acid substitution in the β globin chain causes red cell sickling during deoxygenation, leading to increased rigidity and aggregation in the microcirculation. These changes are reflected by a haemolytic anaemia and episodes of tissue infarction.

Geographical distribution

The sickle cell gene is spread widely throughout Africa and in countries with African immigrant populations; some Mediterranean countries; the Middle East; and parts of India. Screening should not be restricted to people of African origin.

Sickle cell anaemia (homozygous Hb S)

- Anaemia (Hb 60–100 g/l)—Symptoms milder than expected as Hb S has reduced oxygen affinity (that is, gives up oxygen to tissues more easily)
- Sickled cells may be present in blood film—Sickling occurs at oxygen tensions found in venous blood; cyclical sickling episodes
- Reticulocytes—Raised to 10–20%
- Red cells contain ≥80% Hb S (rest is maily fetal Hb)
- Variable haemolysis
- Hand and foot syndrome (dactylitis)
- Intermittent episodes, or crises, characterised by bone pain, worsening anaemia, or pulmonary or neurological disease
- Chronic leg ulcers
- Gall stones

Complications of sickle cell disease

- Hand and foot syndrome—Seen in infancy; painful swelling of digits
- Painful crises—Later in life; generalised bone pain; precipitated by cold, dehydration but often no cause found; self limiting over a few days
- Aplastic crisis—Marrow temporarily hypoplastic; may follow parvovirus infection; profound anaemia; reduced reticulocyte count
- Splenic sequestration crisis—Common in infancy; progressive anaemia; enlargement of spleen
- Hepatic sequestration crisis—Similar to splenic crisis but with sequestration of red cells in liver
- Lung or brain syndromes—Sickling of red cells in pulmonary or cerebral circulation and endothelial damage to cerebral vessels in cerebral circulation
- Infections—Particularly *Streptococcus pneumoniae* and *Haemophilus influenzae*
- Gall stones
- Progressive renal failure
- Chronic leg ulcers
- Recurrent priapism
- Aseptic necrosis of humoral/femoral head
- Chronic osteomyelitis—Sometimes due to *Salmonella typhi*

Clinical features

Sickle cell carriers are not anaemic and have no clinical abnormalities. Patients with sickle cell anaemia have a haemolytic anaemia, with haemoglobin concentration 60-100 g/l and a high reticulocyte count; the blood film shows polychromasia and sickled erythrocytes.

Patients adapt well to their anaemia, and it is the vascular occlusive or sequestration episodes ("crises") that pose the main threat.

Diagnosis

Sickle cell anaemia should be suspected in any patient of an appropriate racial group with a haemolytic anaemia. It can be confirmed by a sickle cell test, although this does not distinguish between heterozygotes and homozygotes. A definitive diagnosis requires haemoglobin electrophoresis and the demonstration of the sickle cell trait in both parents.

Prevention and treatment

Pregnant women in at-risk racial groups should be screened in early pregnancy and, if the woman and her partner are carriers, should be offered either prenatal or neonatal diagnosis. As soon as the diagnosis is established babies should receive penicillin daily and be immunised against *Streptococcus pneumoniae*, *Haemophilus influenzae* type b and *Neisseria meningitidis*. Parents should be warned to seek medical advice on any suspicion of infection.

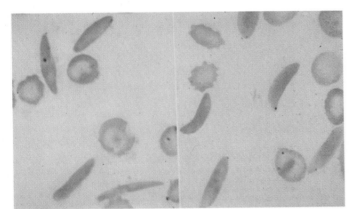

Figure 3.2 Peripheral blood film from patient with sickle cell anaemia showing sickled erythrocytes.

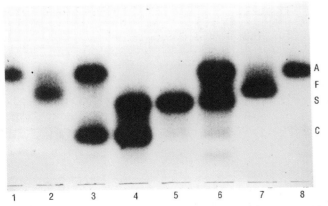

Figure 3.3 Haemoglobin electrophoresis showing (1) normal, (2) newborn, (3) Hb C trait (A-C), (4) Hb SC disease (SC), (5) sickle cell disease (SS), (6) sickle cell trait (A-S), (7) newborn, (8) normal.

Sickling variants

Hb SC disease is characterised by a mild anaemia and fewer crises. Important microvascular complications, however, include retinal damage and blindness, aseptic necrosis of the femoral heads, and recurrent haematuria. The disease is occasionally complicated by pulmonary embolic disease, particularly during and after pregnancy; these episodes

Treatment of major complications of sickle cell disease

- *Hand and foot syndrome*—Hydration; paracetamol
- *Painful crises*—Hydration; analgesia (including graded intravenous analgesics); oxygen (check arterial blood gases); blood cultures; antibiotics
- *Pulmonary infiltrates*—Especially with deterioration in arterial gases, falling platelet count and/or haemoglobin concentration suggesting lung syndrome requires urgent exchange blood transfusion to reduce Hb S level together with oxygenation
- *Splenic sequestration crisis*—Transfusion; splenectomy to prevent recurrence
- *Neurological symptoms*—Immediate exchange transfusion followed by long term transfusion
- *Prevention of crises*—Ongoing trials of cytotoxic agent hydroxyurea show that it raises Hb F level and ameliorates frequency and severity of crises; long term effects unknown

should be treated by immediate exchange transfusion. Patients with Hb SC should have annual ophthalmological surveillance; the retinal vessel proliferation can be controlled with laser treatment. The management of the symptomatic forms of sickle cell β thalassaemia is similar to that of sickle cell anaemia.

The thalassaemias

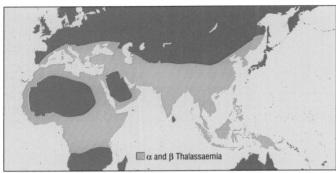

Figure 3.4 Distribution of the thalassaemias (orange area).

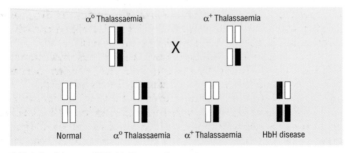

Figure 3.5 Inheritance of Hb H disease (open boxes represent normal α globin genes and black boxes deleted α globin genes).

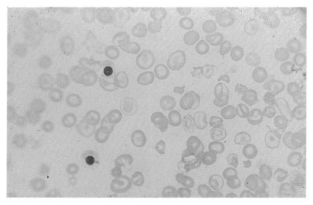

Figure 3.6 Peripheral blood film in homozygous β thalassaemia showing pronounced hypochromia and anisocytosis with nucleated red blood cells.

Classification

The thalassaemias are classified as α or β thalassaemias, depending on which pair of globin chains is synthesised inefficiently. Rarer forms affect both β and δ chain production, δβ thalassaemias.

Distribution

The disease is broadly distributed throughout parts of Africa, the Mediterranean region, the Middle East, the Indian subcontinent, and South East Asia and occurs sporadically in all racial groups. Like sickle cell anaemia, it is thought to be common because carriers have been protected against malaria.

Inheritance

The β thalassaemias result from over 150 different mutations of the β globin genes, which reduce the output of β globin chains, either completely (β° thalassaemia) or partially (β⁺ thalassaemia). They are inherited like sickle cell anaemia; carrier parents have a one in four chance of having a homozygous child. The genetics of the α thalassaemias is more complicated because normal people have two α globin genes on each of their chromosomes 16. If both are lost (α° thalassaemia) no α globin chains are made, whereas if only one of the pair is lost (α⁺ thalassaemia) the output of α globin chains is reduced. Impaired α globin production leads to excess γ or β chains that form unstable and physiologically useless tetramers, γ_4 (Hb Bart's) and β_4 (Hb H). The homozygous state for α° thalassaemia results in the Hb Bart's hydrops syndrome, whereas the inheritance of α° and α⁺ thalassaemia produces Hb H disease.

The β thalassaemias

Heterozygotes for β thalassaemia are asymptomatic, have hypochromic microcytic red cells with a low mean cell haemoglobin and mean cell volume, and have a mean Hb A_2 level of about twice normal. Homozygotes, or those who have inherited a different β thalassaemia gene from both parents, usually develop severe anaemia in the first year of life. This results from a deficiency of β globin

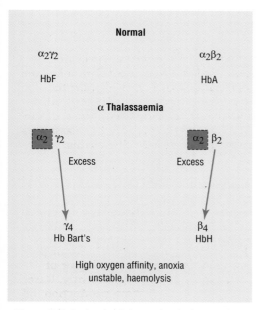

Figure 3.7 Pathophysiology of α thalassaemia.

β Thalassaemia trait (heterozygous carrier)

- Mild hypochromic microcytic anaemia
    Haemoglobin 90–110 g/l
    Mean cell volume 50–70 fl
    Mean corpuscular haemoglobin 20–22 pg
- No clinical features, patients asymptomatic
- Often diagnosed on routine blood count
- Raised Hb A$_2$ level

β Thalassaemia major (homozygous β thalassaemia)

- Severe anaemia
- Blood film
    Pronounced variation in red cell size and shape
    Pale (hypochromic) red cells
    Target cells
    Basophilic stippling
    Nucleated red cells
    Moderately raised reticulocyte count
- Infants are well at birth but develop anaemia in first few months of life when switch occurs from γ to β globin chains
- Progressive splenomegaly; iron loading; proneness to infection

chains; excess α chains precipitate in the red cell precursors leading to their damage, either in the bone marrow or the peripheral blood. Hypertrophy of the ineffective bone marrow leads to skeletal changes, and there is variable hepatosplenomegaly. The Hb F level is always raised. If these children are transfused, the marrow is "switched off," and growth and development may be normal. However, they accumulate iron and may die later from damage to the myocardium, pancreas, or liver. They are also prone to infection and folic acid deficiency. Milder forms of β thalassaemia (thalassaemia intermedia), although not transfusion dependent, are sometimes associated with similar bone changes, anaemia, leg ulcers, and delayed development.

The α thalassaemias

The Hb Bart's hydrops fetalis syndrome is characterised by the stillbirth of a severely oedematous (hydropic) fetus in the second half of pregnancy. Hb H disease is associated with a moderately severe haemolytic anaemia. The carrier states for α° thalassaemia or the homozygous state for α$^+$ thalassaemia result in a mild hypochromic anaemia with normal Hb A$_2$ levels. They can only be distinguished with certainty by DNA analysis in a specialised laboratory. In addition to the distribution mentioned above, α thalassaemia is also seen in European populations in association with mental retardation; the molecular pathology is quite different to the common inherited forms of the condition.

Prevention and treatment

As β thalassaemia is easily identified in heterozygotes, pregnant women of appropriate racial groups should be screened; if a woman is found to be a carrier, her partner should be tested and the couple counselled. Prenatal diagnosis by chorionic villus sampling can be carried out between the 9th and 13th weeks of pregnancy. If diagnosis is established, the patients should be treated by regular blood transfusion with surveillance for hepatitis C and related infections.

To prevent iron overload, overnight infusions of desferrioxamine together with vitamin C should be started, and the patient's serum ferritin and hepatic iron concentrations should be monitored; complications of desferrioxamine include infections with *Yersinia* spp, retinal and acoustic nerve damage, and reduction in growth associated with calcification of the vertebral discs. The place of the oral chelating agent deferiprone (L1) is still under evaluation; though effective, it may cause neutropenia and transient arthritis. Bone marrow transplantation—if appropriate HLA-DR matched siblings are available—may carry a good prognosis if carried out early in life. Treatment with agents designed to raise the production of Hb F is still at the experimental stage.

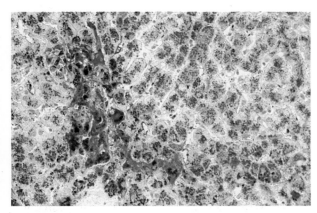

Figure 3.8 Liver biopsy from patient with β thalassaemia showing pronounced iron accumulation.

The α thalassaemias

-α/αα 1α gene deleted
- Asymptomatic
- Minority show reduced mean cell volume and mean corpuscular haemoglobin

-α/-α or αα/- - 2α genes deleted
- Haemoglobin is normal or slightly reduced
- Reduced mean cell volume and mean corpuscular haemoglobin
- No symptoms

- -/-α 3α genes deleted, Hb H disease
- Chronic haemolytic anaemia
- Reduced α chain production with formation of β_4 tetramers (β_4 is termed Hb H)
- Hb H is unstable and precipitates in older red cells
- Haemoglobin is 70–110 g/l, though may be lower
- Reduced mean cell volume and mean corpuscular haemoglobin
- Clinical features: jaundice, hepatosplenomegaly, leg ulcers, gall stones, folate deficiency

- -/- - 4α genes deleted, Hb Bart's hydrops
- No α chains produced
- Mainly γ, forms tetramers (γ_4 = Hb Bart's)
- Intrauterine death or stillborn at 25–40 weeks or dies soon after birth

αα/αα Represents 2α globin genes inherited from each parent
Changes due to α thalassaemia are present from birth unlike in β thalassaemia

In β thalassaemia and Hb H disease progressive splenomegaly or increasing blood requirements, or both, indicate that splenectomy may be beneficial. Patients who undergo splenectomy should be vaccinated against *S pneumoniae*, *H influenzae*, and *N meningitidis* preoperatively and should receive a maintenance dose of oral penicillin indefinitely.

Women with thalassaemia

- Women with the haematological features of thalassaemia trait with normal Hb A_2 levels should be referred to a centre able to identify the different forms of α thalassaemia
- Those with α° thalassaemia trait—if their partners are similarly affected—should be referred for prenatal diagnosis
- This is because the haemoglobin Bart's hydrops syndrome is associated with an increased risk of toxaemia of pregnancy and postpartum bleeding due to a hypertrophied placenta

Red cell enzyme defects

Drugs causing haemolysis in patients with G6PD deficiency

Antimalarials
Primiquine
Pamaquine

Analgesics*
Phenacetin
Acetyl salicylic acid

Others
Sulphonamides
Nalidixic acid
Dapsone

* Probably only at high doses

Red cells have two main metabolic pathways, one burning glucose anaerobically to produce energy, the other generating reduced glutathione to protect against injurious oxidants. Many inherited enzyme defects have been described. Some of those of the energy pathway—for example, pyruvate kinase deficiency—cause haemolytic anaemia; any child with this kind of anaemia from birth should be referred to a centre capable of analysing the major red cell enzymes.

Glucose-6-phosphate dehydrogenase deficiency (G6PD) involves the protective pathway. It affects millions of people worldwide, mainly the same racial groups as are affected by the thalassaemias. Glucose-6-phosphate dehydrogenase deficiency is sex linked and affects males predominantly. It causes neonatal jaundice, sensitivity to fava beans (broad beans), and haemolytic responses to oxidant drugs.

Red cell membrane defects

Further reading

- Davies SC, Wonke B. The management of haemoglobinopathies. *Clin Haematol* 1991;4:361–89.
- Olivieri NF: Iron chelation therapy and thalassemia. In: Kelton JG, Brain M, eds. *Current Therapy in Hematology/Oncology*. 5th ed. Philadelphia: Decker, 1995:80–9.
- Weatherall DJ. The Thalassemias. In: Stamatoyannopoulos G, Nienhuis AW, Majerus PW, Varmus H, eds. *The Molecular Basis of Blood Diseases*. 2nd ed. Philadelphia: Saunders, 1994:157–95.
- Weatherall DJ. The thalassemias. In: Beutler E, Lichtman MA, Coller BS, Kipps TJ, eds. *Williams Hematology*. 5th ed. New York: McGraw-Hill (in press).

The red cell membrane is a complex sandwich of proteins that are required to maintain the integrity of the cell. There are many inherited defects of the membrane proteins, some of which cause haemolytic anaemia. Hereditary spherocytosis is due to a structural change that makes the cells more leaky. It is particularly important to identify this disease because it can be "cured" by splenectomy. There are many rare inherited varieties of elliptical or oval red cells, some associated with chronic haemolysis and response to splenectomy. A child with a chronic haemolytic anaemia with abnormally shaped red cells should always be referred for expert advice.

Other hereditary anaemias

Other anaemias with an important inherited component include Fanconi's anaemia (hypoplastic anaemia with skeletal deformities), Blackfan-Diamond anaemia (red cell aplasia), and several forms of congenital dyserythropoietic anaemia.

4 POLYCYTHAEMIA, PRIMARY (ESSENTIAL) THROMBOCYTHAEMIA AND MYELOFIBROSIS

Maria Messinezy, T C Pearson

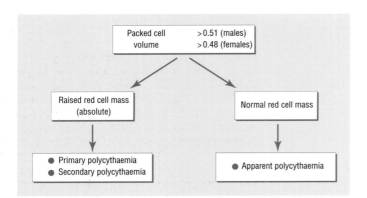

Primary polycythaemia (polycythaemia rubra vera), primary (or essential) thrombocythaemia, and myelofibrosis are all clonal disorders originating from a single aberrant neoplastic stem cell in the bone marrow. They are generally diseases of middle or older age and have or may develop features in common, including a small potential for transforming to acute leukaemia. Myelofibrosis may arise *de novo* or result from progression of primary polycythaemia or primary thrombocythaemia. Treatment of primary polycythaemia and primary thrombocythaemia can greatly influence prognosis, hence the importance of diagnosing these rare disorders. They need to be distinguished from other types of polycythaemia (secondary polycythaemia, apparent polycythaemia) and other causes of a raised platelet count (secondary or reactive thrombocytosis), whose prognosis is different.

Polycythaemia

Symptoms and signs of primary polycythaemia

- Stroke
- Transient ischaemic attack
- Digital ischaemia
- Headache
- Mental clouding
- Facial plethora
- Pruritus
- Bleeding (including gastrointestinal tract)
- Gout

Palpable splenomegaly is present in less than half of patients with primary polycythaemia, but when present it reliably distinguishes primary polycythaemia from the other polycythaemias

---

Aims of treatment of primary polycythaemia

- To reduce packed cell volume to < 0.45 (by regular venesection)
- To reduce platelet count to < 400×10⁹/l (by daily hydroxyurea)

The packed cell volume, rather than the haemoglobin concentration, is the indicator of polycythaemia. A raised packed cell volume (> 0·51 in males, > 0·48 in females) needs to be confirmed on a specimen taken without venous occlusion. Patients with a persistently raised packed cell volume should be referred to a haematologist for measurement of red cell mass by radionuclide labelling of the red cells. Red cell mass is best expressed as the percentage difference between the measured value and that predicted from the patient's height and weight (derived from tables).

Red cell mass more than 25% above the predicted value constitutes real or absolute polycythaemia, of which there are two types: primary and secondary. When the packed cell volume is raised but the red cell mass is not, the condition is known as apparent polycythaemia.

Primary polycythaemia

Presentation can be incidental but is classically associated with a history of occlusive vascular lesions (stroke, transient ischaemic attack, ischaemic digits), headache, mental clouding, facial redness, itching, abnormal bleeding, or gout.

Initial laboratory investigations—A raised white cell count (> 10×10⁹/l neutrophils) or a raised platelet count (> 400×10⁹/l) suggest primary polycythaemia, especially if both are raised in the absence of an obvious cause, such as infection or carcinoma. Serum ferritin concentration should be determined as iron deficiency may mask a raised packed cell volume, resulting in a missed diagnosis.

Specialist investigations—Red cell mass should be determined to confirm absolute polycythaemia, and secondary polycythaemia should be excluded. Most patients with primary polycythaemia have a low serum erythropoietin concentration. If the spleen is not palpable then splenic sizing (ultrasonography) should be performed to look for

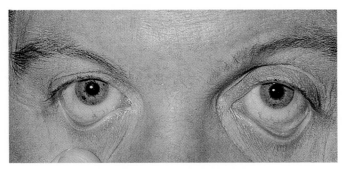

Figure 4.2 Facial redness in patient with primary polycythaemia.

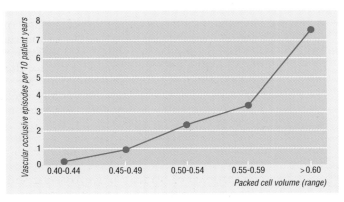

Figure 4.3 Packed cell volume versus incidence of thrombotic events.

Median survival in primary polycythaemia

- Untreated patients—18 months, death being due mainly to vascular occlusion (especially strokes)
- Treated patients—10 to15 years

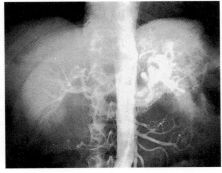

Figure 4.4 Angiogram in patient with hypernephroma leading to secondary polycythaemia.

Causes of secondary polycythaemia

- Hypoxaemia—for example, chronic lung disease, cyanotic congenital heart disease, and sleep apnoea
- Renal—for example, hypernephroma, polycystic kidney disease, and post renal transplant
- Miscellaneous—for example, hepatoma, cerebellar haemangioma, raised oxygen affinity haemoglobin

Investigations in suspected secondary polycythaemia

Routine
- Arterial oxygen saturation (pulse oximetry)
- Renal, hepatic, and splenic ultrasound

Specialist
- Serum erythropoietin
- Oxygen affinity of haemoglobin (p50)
- Sleep study (if clinically indicated)

enlargement. Bone marrow chromosomal analysis may show changes that establish clonality which would be in favour of a primary marrow disorder such as primary polycythaemia. Abnormal features of erythroid colony growth in culture from peripheral blood can support the diagnosis.

Treatment—Traditional treatment using the marrow suppressant effect of radioactive phosphorus (^{32}P) has been largely superseded because of the additional risk of inducing malignancies such as acute leukaemia in later life. It is still useful, however, in elderly people and when venous access or patient attendance or compliance is poor. Repeated venesection to maintain the packed cell volume at <0.45 has become the mainstay of treatment. At this volume the risk of thrombotic episodes is much reduced. Venesection has to be frequent at first but is eventually needed only every six to 10 weeks in most patients. Concurrent cytotoxic therapy to control the platelet count (<400×10⁹/l) is necessary. Hydroxyurea (0.5-1.5 g daily) is recommended for this purpose and is not thought to have a pronounced leukaemogenic potential. Low dose intermittent oral busulphan is often more convenient in elderly people, in whom potential side effects may be more acceptable.

Progression—Long survival (>10 years) of the treated patient has revealed a 20% incidence of transformation to myelofibrosis and about 5% to acute leukaemia. The incidence of leukaemia is further increased in those who have transformed to myelofibrosis and those treated with ^{32}P or high dose cytotoxic agents.

Secondary polycythaemia

Many causes of secondary polycythaemia have been identified, the commonest being hypoxaemia (arterial saturation <92%) and renal lesions. Investigations are designed to determine the underlying cause to which the polycythaemia is secondary.

Treatment is aimed at removing the underlying cause when practicable. In hypoxaemia—in which the risk of vascular occlusion is much less pronounced than in primary polycythaemia—venesection is usually undertaken only in those with a very high packed cell volume. Reduction to packed cell volume 0.50-0.52 may result in an improvement of cardiopulmonary function. At this level the harmful effects of increased viscosity no longer outweigh the oxygen carrying benefits of a raised packed cell volume. In polycythaemia associated with renal lesions or other tumours, the packed cell volume should generally be reduced to <0.45.

Apparent polycythaemia

In apparent polycythaemia red cell mass is not increased, and there is no evidence of primary or secondary polycythaemia. Some association exists with smoking, increased alcohol intake, obesity, diuretics, and hypertension.

The need for treatment is uncertain. Lowering the packed cell volume by venesection is undertaken only in patients who have increased risk of vascular occlusion for other reasons, or whose packed cell volume is >0.54. On follow up one third of patients revert spontaneously to normal packed cell volume.

Since some patients with apparent polycythaemia may be at an early

This supersedes older nomenclature including terms such as:

- Pseudo, spurious, or relative polycythaemia
- Stress erythrocytosis
- Gaisbock's syndrome

stage of progression to absolute polycythaemia, investigations for primary or secondary polycythaemia are relevant even when the red cell mass is normal.

Primary (essential) thrombocythaemia

Differential diagnosis of a raised platelet count

- Reactive thrombocytosis due to:
  Infection
  Malignancy
  Chronic inflammatory bowel disease
  Hyposplenism
  Bleeding
- Primary thrombocythaemia
- Primary polycythaemia
- Myelofibrosis
- Myelodysplasia

If there is palpable splenomegaly a raised platelet count is much more likely to be due to primary thrombocythaemia than to reactive thrombocytosis

---

Exclusion requirements for diagnosing primary thrombocythaemia

- Reactive thrombocytosis—History and general clinical examination may reveal underlying conditions such as infection or malignancy to which the raised platelet count may be secondary
- Primary polycythaemia should be suspected if the packed cell volume is raised (or the rise is masked by coexisting iron deficiency)
- Myelofibrosis (teardrop red cells, nucleated red cells and immature white cells—for example, myelocytes—in the peripheral blood, marrow fibrosis on trephine). A raised platelet count may be an early feature
- Myelodysplasia (dysplastic peripheral blood and bone marrow cells, abnormal karyotype). Some patients have a raised platelet count

---

Gangrene of the toes in the presence of good peripheral pulses and a raised platelet count strongly suggests primary thrombocythaemia

---

Like primary polycythaemia and myelofibrosis, primary thrombocythaemia is one of the group of clonal conditions known as the myeloproliferative disorders.

A persisting platelet count $> 600 \times 10^9/l$ is the central diagnostic feature. But other causes of raised platelet count need to be excluded before a diagnosis of primary thrombocythaemia can be made.

Laboratory investigations

Investigations may reveal other causes of raised platelet count. Apart from a full blood count and blood film they should also include erythrocyte sedimentation rate, serum concentrations of C reactive protein and serum ferritin; bone marrow aspirate, trephine and cytogenetic analysis (this is generally normal, but abnormalities may favour a diagnosis of myelodysplasia, and, very occasionally, the Philadelphia chromosome is present).

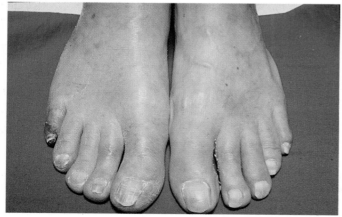

Figure 4.5 Toe gangrene in patient with essential thrombocythaemia.

Presentation and prognosis

Thirty to fifty per cent of patients with primary thrombocythaemia have microvascular occlusive events—for example, burning pain in extremities (erythromelalgia) or digital ischaemia—major vascular occlusive events, or haemorrhage at presentation. These are most pronounced in elderly people in whom the risk of cerebrovascular accident, myocardial infarction, or other vascular occlusion is very high in untreated patients. The risk in young patients is lower, though major life threatening events have been described. Transformation to myelofibrosis or acute leukaemia may occur in the long term in a minority of patients.

Treatment and survival

All patients should receive daily low dose aspirin, unless contra-indicated because of bleeding or peptic ulceration. This reduces the risk of vascular occlusion but may increase the risk of haemorrhage, particularly at very high platelet counts.

Reduction of the platelet count by cytotoxic agents (daily hydroxyurea or intermittent low dose busulphan in elderly people) reduces the incidence of vascular complications and appreciably improves survival in older patients (from about three years in untreated to 10 years or more in treated patients). Newer drugs, such as anagrelide or interferon alfa, are under investigation.

The value of these cytotoxic agents in young patients is uncertain-particularly in the face of a possible leukaemogenic risk made worse by the prospect of many years of treatment. Clinical trials comparing the effects of different cytotoxic agents and looking at the possibility of not lowering the platelet count in young asymptomatic patients are planned.

> The risk of occlusive vascular lesions is very small in reactive thrombocytosis but high in primary thrombocythaemia

Idiopathic myelofibrosis (primary)

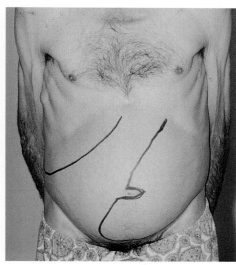

Figure 4.6 Massive splenomegaly in patient with myelofibrosis

The main features are bone marrow fibrosis, extramedullary haemopoiesis (that is, production of blood cells within organs such as the spleen), splenomegaly, and leucoerythroblastic blood picture (immature red and white cells in the peripheral blood). Good evidence exists that the fibroblast proliferation is secondary (reactive) and not part of the clonal process. Idiopathic myelofibrosis needs to be distinguished from causes of secondary myelofibrosis (see below).

Presentation

Idiopathic myelofibrosis (primary) may have been present for many years before diagnosis. Patients could have had previous undiagnosed primary polycythaemia or thrombocythaemia. The absence of an easily palpable spleen is rare. The main presenting features are abdominal mass (splenomegaly), weight loss (hypermetabolic state), anaemia, fatigue, and bleeding.

Laboratory investigations

The blood count is variable. In the initial "proliferative phase" red cell production may be normal or even increased. About half of presenting patients may have a raised white cell count or platelet count (absence of Philadelphia chromosome will distinguish from chronic myeloid leukaemia). As the bone marrow becomes more fibrotic, the classic "cytopenic phase" supervenes the occurence.

Laboratory investigation of idiopathic myelofibrosis (primary)

Peripheral blood
- Normochromic anaemia (teardrop red cells)
- Nucleated red cells and immature neutrophils
- Thrombocytopenia and large abnormal platelets

Bone marrow examination
- "Dry" or "blood tap" on aspiration
- Biopsy (trephine) shows increased fibrous tissue, with variable amounts of cellular marrow in between (megakaryocytes prominent)

Indications for splenectomy in myelofibrosis

- Frequent blood transfusion
- Troublesome thrombocytopenia
- Large painful spleen

Secondary myelofibrosis

This is not a clonal myeloproliferative disorder but a reaction to other diseases. The diagnosis is based on discovering associated disease:
- Primary marrow malignancy—for example, myelo-dysplasia, myeloma
- Secondary metastatic carcinoma
- Chronic infections—for example, tuberculosis

Progression and management

Survival varies, with a median of two to four years. It may be much longer in patients who are asymptomatic at presentation.

Supportive blood transfusion may be needed for anaemic patients. Cytotoxic agents may be useful in the proliferative phase to suppress the bone marrow. Splenectomy will improve the quality of life (though not the prognosis) by reducing the need for transfusion and the occurrence thrombocytopenia. Operative morbidity and mortality can be high when the splenomegaly is gross. Low dose irradiation of the spleen may be helpful in frail patients.

Death can be due to haemorrhage, infection, cardiac failure, or transformation to acute leukaemia. Portal hypertension with varices, iron overload from blood transfusion, and compression of vital structures by extramedullary haemopoietic masses may also contribute to morbidity.

We thank Monica Nestor for secretarial help. The graph was adapted, with permission, from the *Lancet* (Pearson TC *et al*. Vascular occlusive episodes and venous haematocrit in primary proliferative polycythaemia. 1978;ii:1219-22). The photographs of facial plethora and splenomegaly are reproduced with permission from *Clinical Haematology Illustrated* (A V Hoffbrand, J E Pettit), Edinburgh: Churchill Livingstone, 1987.

5 Chronic myeloid leukaemia

John Goldman

Chronic myeloid leukaemia is a clonal malignant myeloproliferative disorder believed to originate in a single abnormal haemopoietic stem cell. The progeny of this abnormal stem cell proliferate over months or years such that, by the time the leukaemia is diagnosed, the number of leucocytes is greatly increased in the peripheral blood. Normal blood cell production is almost completely replaced by leukaemia cells, which, however, still function almost normally.

Chronic myeloid leukaemia has an annual incidence of 1 to 1·5 per 100 000 of the population (in the United Kingdom about 700 new cases each year), with no clear geographical variation.

Presentation may be at any age, but the peak incidence is at age 40-60 years, with a slight male predominance. This leukaemia is very rare in children.

Most cases of chronic myeloid leukaemia occur sporadically. The only known predisposing factor is irradiation, as shown by studies of Japanese survivors of the atomic bomb and in patients who received radiotherapy for ankylosing spondylitis.

The clinical course of chronic myeloid leukaemia can be divided into a "stable" or chronic phase and an advanced phase, the latter covering both accelerated and blastic phases. Most patients present with chronic phase disease, which lasts on average four to five years. In about two thirds of patients the chronic phase transforms gradually into an accelerated phase, characterised by a moderate increase in blast cells, increasing anaemia or thrombocytosis, or other features not compatible with chronic phase disease. After a variable number of months this accelerated phase progresses to frank acute blastic transformation. The remaining one third of patients move abruptly from chronic phase to an acute blastic phase (or blastic crisis) without an intervening phase of acceleration.

Clinical features in patients with chronic myeloid leukaemia at diagnosis

Common
- Fatigue
- Weight loss
- Sweating
- Anaemia
- Haemorrhage—for example, easy bruising, discrete ecchymoses
- Splenomegaly with or without hepatomegaly

Rare
- Splenic infarction
- Leucostasis
- Gout
- Retinal haemorrhages
- Priapism
- Fever

Survival from chronic myeloid leukaemia

- The average survival from diagnosis is five to six years, but the range is wide
- Occasionally patients die within one year of diagnosis
- About 3% of patients may live more than 15 years without radical therapy

Pathogenesis

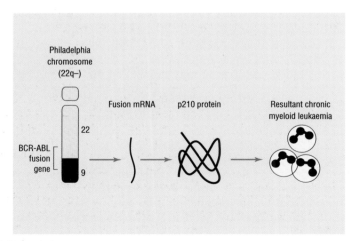

Figure 5.1 Formation of the Philadelphia chromosome resulting in a BCR-ABL fusion gene that generates a fusion protein (p210) responsible for the chronic myeloid leukaemia phenotype.

All leukaemia cells in patients with chronic myeloid leukaemia contain a specific cytogenetic marker, described originally in 1960 by workers in Philadelphia and known consequently as the Philadelphia or Ph chromosome.

The Ph chromosome is derived from a normal 22 chromosome that has lost part of its long arm as a result of a balanced reciprocal translocation of DNA involving one of the 22 and one of the 9 chromosomes. The translocation is usually referred to as t(9;22)(q34;q11). Thus the Ph chromosome (22q−) appears somewhat shorter than its normal counterpart and the 9q+ somewhat longer than the normal 9.

The Ph chromosome carries a specific fusion gene known as BCR-ABL, which results from juxtaposition of the ABL proto-oncogene (from chromosome 9) with part of the BCR gene on chromosome 22. This fusion gene is expressed as a specific messenger RNA (mRNA), which in turn generates a protein called p210. This protein perturbs stem cell function, resulting in the chronic phase of chronic myeloid leukaemia, although the exact mechanism remains unclear.

Researchers are working to inactivate the BCR-ABL gene and thereby reverse the leukaemic phenotype in chronic myeloid leukaemia cells.

Chronic phase disease

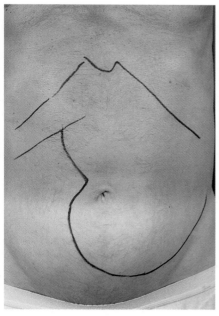

Figure 5.2 Patient with massive splenomegaly in chronic phase chronic myeloid leukaemia.

> The spleen may be greatly enlarged before onset of symptoms. Treatment that reduces leucocyte count to normal usually restores the spleen to normal size

Usual peripheral blood findings in chronic myeloid leukaemia at diagnosis

- Raised white blood cell count $(30-400\times10^9/l)$.
  Differential shows:
    Granulocytes at all stages of development
    Increased numbers of basophils and eosinophils
    Blast (primitive) cells (maximum 10%) - never present in the blood of normal people
- Haemoglobin concentration may be reduced; red cell morphology is usually unremarkable; nucleated (immature) red cells may be present
- Platelet count may be raised $(300-600\times10^9/l)$

Investigations to confirm suspected chronic myeloid leukaemia

Routine
- Full blood count including blood film
- Neutrophil alkaline phosphatase
- Urea, electrolytes
- Serum lactate dehydrogenase
- Bone marrow aspirate (degree of cellularity, chromosome analysis)

Optional
- Bone marrow trephine biopsy (extent of fibrosis)
- BCR-ABL chimeric gene by fluorescence in situ hybridisation or by polymerase chain reaction
- Vitamin B_{12} and B_{12} binding capacity
- HLA typing for patient and family members

Presentation

The characteristic symptoms at presentation include fatigue, weight loss, sweating, anaemia, haemorrhage or purpura, and the sensation of a mass in the left upper abdominal quadrant (spleen). Often the disease is detected as a result of routine blood tests performed for unrelated reasons, and a fifth of patients are totally asymptomatic at the time of diagnosis. The spleen may be greatly enlarged before onset of symptoms. Treatment that reduces the leucocyte count to normal usually restores the spleen to normal size. Much rarer features at presentation include non-specific fever, lymphadenopathy, visual disturbances due to leucostasis (a form of hyperviscosity caused by an extremely high white cell count) or retinal haemorrhages, splenic pain due to infarction, gout, and occasionally priapism.

The commonest physical sign at diagnosis is an enlarged spleen, which may vary from being just palpable at the left costal margin to filling the whole left side of the abdomen and extending towards the right iliac fossa. The liver may be enlarged, with a soft, rather ill defined lower edge. Spontaneous and excessive bruising in response to minor trauma is common.

Diagnosis

The diagnosis of chronic myeloid leukaemia in chronic phase can be made from study of the peripheral blood film, but the marrow is usually examined for confirmation.

Marrow examination shows increased cellularity. The distribution of immature leucocytes resembles that seen in the blood film. Red cell production is relatively reduced. Megakaryocytes, the cells giving rise to platelets, are plentiful but may be smaller than usual.

Cytogenetic study of marrow shows the presence of the Ph chromosome in all dividing cells.

The patient's blood concentrations of urea and electrolytes are usually normal at diagnosis, whereas the lactate dehydrogenase is usually raised. Serum urate concentration may be raised.

Management

After diagnosis the first priority is a frank discussion with the patient. It is now customary to use the term leukaemia in this discussion and to explain to the patient that he or she may expect to live for several years with a near normal lifestyle. The clinician should explain the propensity of the disease to progress to an advanced phase. The choice of treatment with interferon alfa or hydroxyurea should be discussed.

If chronic myeloid leukaemia is diagnosed in pregnancy the woman should have the chance to continue to term. Chronic myeloid leukaemia has no adverse effect on pregnancy and pregnancy has no adverse effect on the leukaemia.

The clinician may wish to mention at this stage the two ongoing Medical Research Council trials on chronic myeloid leukaemia. Patient information booklets produced by BACUP (British Association of Cancer United Patients) and by the Leukaemia Research Fund are extremely valuable as many patients will not retain all that is said at this first interview.

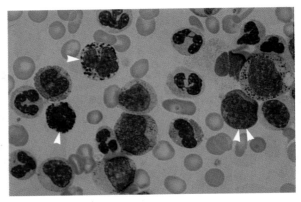

Figure 5.3 Peripheral blood film from patient with chronic myeloid leukaemia showing many mature granulocytes, including two basophils (arrow); a blast cell is prominent (double arrow).

> Younger men should be offered cryopreservation of semen if necessary

Treatment with hydroxyurea

- Hydroxyurea inhibits the enzyme ribonucleotide reductase and acts specifically on cells of the myeloid series—that is, neutrophils, eosinophils, basophils, etc
- It is useful for rapid reduction of the leucocyte count in newly diagnosed patients
- Many haematologists start treatment with hydroxyurea then switch to interferon alfa once the patient's symptoms are relieved and the leucocyte count is restored to normal
- Hydroxyurea is also valuable for controlling chronic phase disease in patients who cannot tolerate interferon alfa
- It is usually started at 2·0 g daily by mouth; the usual maintenance dose is 1·0-1·5 g daily, titrated against the leucocyte count
- Treatment with hydroxyurea does not eradicate cells with the Ph chromosome
- Side effects are rare but include rashes, mouth ulceration, and gastrointestinal symptoms. The drug causes macrocytosis and megaloblastoid changes in the marrow

Treatment with busulphan

- Busulphan is an alkylating agent
- It is now reserved for chronic myeloid leukaemia resistant to hydroxyurea or in patients with poor compliance
- Prolonged or excessive dosage may lead to skin pigmentation, pulmonary fibrosis, and marrow aplasia

Interferon alfa—Interferon alfa is a member of a family of naturally occurring glycoproteins with antiviral and antiproliferative actions. It is probably the drug of choice for managing chronic myeloid leukaemia in the chronic phase. Interferon alfa restores spleen size and blood counts to normal in 70-80% of patients. Of great interest is that 10-20% of patients achieve a major reduction or complete disappearance of cells with the Ph chromosome from their bone marrow (disappearance indicates complete remission). Interferon alfa initially causes flu-like symptoms, but these usually subside. Other more persistent side effects include anorexia, weight loss, depression, alopecia, rashes, neuropathies, autoimmune disorders, and thrombocytopenia. Toxicity leads to discontinuation in about a fifth of patients.

Allogeneic bone marrow transplantation—Patients under the age of 60 years who have siblings with identical HLA typing may be offered treatment by high dose cytoreduction (chemotherapy and radiotherapy) followed by transplantation of donor bone marrow. With typical family size in western Europe, about 30% of patients will have matched sibling donors. An appreciable mortality is associated with this approach, and in general, older patients (aged 40-60) fare less well than younger patients. Nevertheless the projected cure rate after allogeneic bone marrow transplantation is about 60%.

Autologous stem cell transplantation—For patients up to the age of 65 years for whom an allograft is excluded, autografting may be considered. For this purpose haemopoietic stem cells are collected from the patient's blood or marrow and cryopreserved. The patient then receives high dose cytoreductive chemotherapy, followed by reinfusion of the thawed stem cells. The morbidity and mortality associated with autografting are much lower than those associated with allografting, but autografting has no potential to cure. It probably prolongs life by one or two years in some cases.

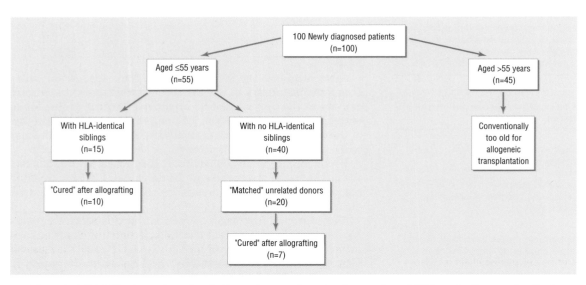

Figure 5.4 Eligibility for and results of allogeneic transplantation for unselected 100 newly diagnosed patients.

Advanced phase disease

Criteria for advanced phase disease

- Increasing splenomegaly despite full doses of cytotoxic drugs
- Rapid white blood cell doubling time
- White blood cell count poorly responsive to full doses of cytotoxic drugs
- Anaemia or thrombocytopenia unresponsive to cytotoxic drugs
- Persistent thrombocytosis ($>1000 \times 10^9$/l)
- $>10\%$ Blasts in peripheral blood or marrow
- $>20\%$ Blasts plus promyelocytes in blood or marrow
- Acquisition of "non-random" chromosomal changes in addition to presence of Philadelphia chromosome
- Development of myelofibrosis

At times the advanced phase can be difficult to distinguish from the chronic phase and can be diagnosed with confidence only in retrospect

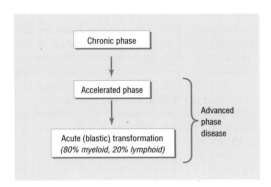

Figure 5.5 Progression of chronic myeloid leukaemia showing progression to blastic phase.

Presentation

Advanced phase disease may be diagnosed incidentally as a result of a blood test at a routine clinic visit. Alternatively the patient may have excessive sweating, persistent fever, or otherwise unexplained symptoms of anaemia, splenic enlargement or splenic infarction, haemorrhage, or bone pain. In most cases the blast crisis is myeloid (that is, resembling acute myeloid leukaemia), and in a fifth of cases lymphoid blast crisis occurs.

Occasionally patients progress to a myelofibrotic phase of the disease, in which intense marrow fibrosis predominates, blast cells proliferate less aggressively, and the clinical picture is characterised by splenomegaly and pancytopenia consequent on marrow failure.

Management

Patients in advanced phase may benefit from introduction of hydroxyurea or busulphan if they have not previously received these. Splenectomy may be useful to improve thrombocytopenia or symptoms due to splenomegaly. Patients in a blastic phase may be treated by combination chemotherapy, though the possibility of treating localised pain or resistant splenomegaly by radiotherapy should not be forgotten. For those with myeloid transformations drugs suitable for treating acute myeloid leukaemia will control the leukaemic proliferation for a time. About 30% of patients will achieve a second chronic phase compatible with a normal lifestyle for months or years. Patients with lymphoid transformations should be treated with drugs appropriate to adult acute lymphoblastic leukaemia. Second chronic phase may be achieved in 40-60% of cases, more commonly in those who had a short interval from diagnosis to transformation. Patients restored to second chronic phase should receive craniospinal prophylaxis comprising five or six intrathecal injections of methotrexate. Cranial or craniospinal irradiation is probably not indicated.

6   THE ACUTE LEUKAEMIAS

R J Liesner, A H Goldstone

Acute leukaemia is a clonal (that is, derived from a single cell) malignant disorder affecting all age groups from infancy to old age. It is characterised by the accumulation of abnormal white blood cells in the bone marrow which replace normal marrow tissue, including haemopoietic precursor cells. This results in bone marrow failure and peripheral blood involvement. Infiltration of various organs is also a feature of some forms of leukaemia.

In most cases the aetiology is not obvious, but some constitutional and acquired disorders do predispose to acute leukaemia. In the past 40 years advances in the treatment of acute leukaemia have improved the chance of cure from virtually zero to 20-75%, depending on age and type of leukaemia. This has largely been the result of clinical trials—many of which are still ongoing—and the development and continued improvements in bone marrow transplantation.

Aetiological factors in acute leukaemia

- Unknown (usually)
- Hereditary
  Down's syndrome
  Bloom's syndrome
  Fanconi's anaemia
  Ataxia telangiectasia
  Kleinfelter's syndrome
  Osteogenesis imperfecta
  Wiskott-Aldrich syndrome
  Leukaemia in siblings
- Chemicals
  Chronic benzene exposure
  Alkylating agents (chlorambucil, melphalan)
- Radiation
- Predisposing haematological diseases (myeloproliferative disorders, myelodysplasia, and aplastic anaemia).
- Viruses (HTLV-I causing adult T cell leukaemia/lymphoma)

Classification

Acute leukaemia is subdivided into (A) acute lymphoblastic leukaemia, in which the abnormal proliferation is in the lymphoid progenitor cells (that is, immature lymphocytes) and (B) acute myeloid leukaemia, which involves the myeloid lineages (that is, cells from which neutrophils, eosinophils, monocytes, basophils, megakaryocytes, etc are derived). The distinction between the two leukaemias is based on morphological, cytochemical, and immunological differences and is of paramount importance as the treatment and prognosis are usually different.

Both acute lymphoblastic leukaemia and acute myeloid leukaemia are further subdivided on the basis of morphological criteria: acute lymphoblastic leukaemia into FAB (French-American-British) subtypes L1, L2, and L3 and acute myeloid leukaemia into FAB subtypes M0 to M7.

On the basis of surface antigen expression acute lymphoblastic leukaemia is divided into T cell lineage and B cell lineage. B cell lineage is further subdivided: early B precursor acute lymphoblastic leukaemia is the most immature and is negative for the common acute lymphoblastic leukaemia antigen (CD10); common acute lymphoblastic leukaemia and pre-B cell acute lymphoblastic leukaemia are more mature and are CD10 positive; and B cell acute lymphoblastic leukaemia is the most mature and is the only one to express surface immunoglobulin. Little correlation exists between morphological subtype and immunophenotype or prognosis in acute lymphoblastic leukaemia, except that L3 morphology is almost exclusively found in B cell acute lymphoblastic leukaemia.

FAB* classification of acute myeloid leukaemia

M0	Acute myeloid leukaemia with minimal evidence of myeloid differentiation
M1	Acute myeloblastic leukaemia without maturation
M2	Acute myeloblastic leukaemia with maturation
M3	Acute promyelocytic leukaemia
M4	Acute myelomonocytic leukaemia
M5	Acute monocytic/monoblastic leukaemia
M6	Acute erythroleukaemia
M7	Acute megakaryoblastic leukaemia

*French-American-British

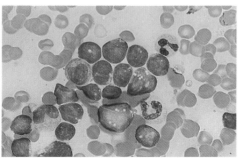

Figure 6.1 Blood film of patient with acute lymphoblastic leukaemia.

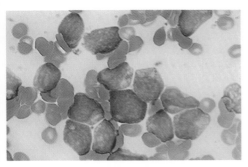

Figure 6.2 Blood film of patient with acute myeloid leukaemia.

In acute myeloid leukaemia immunophenotyping may not help to distinguish between leukaemias of the myeloid (M0 to M3), the myelomonocytic (M4), and the monocytic (M5) lineages, and special cytochemical stains are usually used to support morphological findings. In erythroleukaemia (M6) and megakaryoblastic leukaemia (M7), however, the surface antigen expression is often diagnostic.

Incidence

> Acute lymphoblastic leukaemia is slightly more common among males than females

> Acute myeloid leukaemia is equally common among males and females

Acute lymphoblastic leukaemia

Acute lymphoblastic leukaemia is commonest in the age range 2-10 years with a peak at 3-4 years. The incidence then decreases with increasing age, though there is a secondary rise after 40 years. In children it is the most common malignant disease and accounts for 85% of childhood leukaemia.

Acute myeloid leukaemia

Acute myeloid leukaemia accounts for 10-15% of childhood leukaemia but is the commonest leukaemia of adulthood, particularly as chronic myeloproliferative disorders and preleukaemic conditions such as myelodysplasia usually progress to acute myeloid leukaemia rather than acute lymphoblastic leukaemia. The incidence increases with age, and the median age at presentation is 60 years.

Presentation

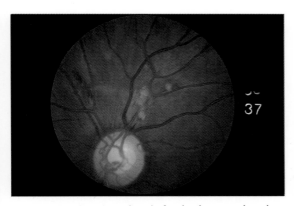

Figure 6.3 Infiltration of optic fundus by acute lymphoblastic leukaemia.

Acute leukaemia is always serious and life threatening, and all patients suspected of having this condition should be immediately referred for urgent assessment.

Common symptoms and signs at presentation result from bone marrow failure or organ infiltration. Anaemia can result in pallor, lethargy, and dyspnoea. Neutropenia results in infections of the mouth, throat, skin, or perianal region. Thrombocytopenia may present as spontaneous bruising, menorrhagia, bleeding from venepuncture sites, gingival bleeding, or prolonged nose bleeds.

A common presenting feature resulting from organ infiltration in childhood acute lymphoblastic leukaemia is bone pain, but acute lymphoblastic leukaemia can also present with superficial lymphadenopathy, abdominal distension due to abdominal lymphadenopathy and hepatosplenomegaly, respiratory embarrassment due to a large mediastinal mass, testicular enlargement, or a meningeal syndrome. Gum hypertrophy and skin infiltration are more commonly seen in acute myeloid than in acute lymphoblastic leukaemia.

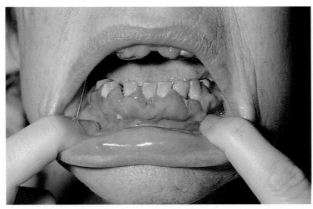

Figure 6.4 Severe gum swelling at presentation in acute myeloid leukaemia M5.

Investigations

Differential diagnosis of acute leukaemia

- If lymphadenopathy—Infections such as infectious mononucleosis or lymphoma
- If hepatosplenomegaly—Myeloproliferative or lymphoproliferative disorder, myelodysplasia, metabolic, storage or autoimmune disorders (rarely, tropical disease—eg visceral leishmaniasis)
- If no peripheral leukaemic blasts but pancytopenia—Aplastic anaemia or infiltrated bone marrow involvement from non-haemopoietic small round cell tumour
- Myelodysplasia
- Lymphoblastic lymphoma—Lymphomatous presentation with <25% of blasts in the marrow (distinction may be arbitrary as treatment may be the same)

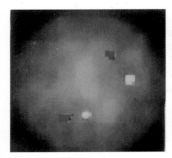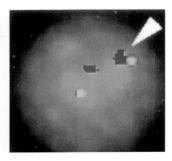

Figure 6.5 Interphase fluorescence in situ hybridisation using probes for BCR and ABL genes. Left: Normal cell showing two red dots (two normal copies of BCR) and two yellow dots (two normal copies of ABL). Right: Cell from child with Ph chromosome positive acute lymphoblastic leukaemia with translocation of chromosomes 9 and 22.

Full blood count usually but not invariably shows reduced haemoglobin concentration and platelet count. The white cell count can vary from $<1.0\times10^9/l$ to $>200\times10^9/l$, and the differential white cell count is often abnormal, with neutropenia and the presence of blast cells. The anaemia is a normochromic, normocytic anaemia, and the thrombocytopenia may be severe (platelet count $<10\times10^9/l$).

Coagulation screening may yield abnormal results, particularly in promyelocytic leukaemia (acute myeloid leukaemia M3) when granules from the leukaemic blasts can have procoagulant activity and trigger a consumptive coagulopathy.

Biochemical screening is particularly important if the leucocyte count is very high, when there may be evidence of renal impairment and hyperuricaemia.

Chest radiography is mandatory to exclude the presence of a mediastinal mass, which is present in up to 70% of patients with T cell acute lymphoblastic leukaemia. In childhood acute lymphoblastic leukaemia lytic bone lesions may also be seen.

Bone marrow aspiration with or without trephination is essential to confirm acute leukaemia. It is usually hypercellular with a predominance of immature (blast) cells.

Immunophenotyping of the antigens present on the bone marrow or peripheral blasts is the most reliable method of determining whether the leukaemia is lymphoid or myeloid, and cytochemistry helps to confirm myeloid or monocytic origin.

Cytogenetics and molecular studies often detect abnormalities within the leukaemic clone that can have diagnostic or prognostic value-for example, the Philadelphia chromosome, which is the product of a translocation between chromosomes 9 and 22, the presence of which confers a very poor prognosis in cases of acute lymphoblastic leukaemia.

Lumbar puncture with cerebrospinal fluid cytospin is an important initial staging investigation to detect leukaemic cells in the cerebrospinal fluid, indicating involvement of the central nervous system.

Management

Management of acute leukaemia

- Immediate (same day) referral to specialist
- Prompt diagnosis
- Early treatment
- Intensive supportive care
- Systemic chemotherapy
- Treatment directed at central nervous system (in children and in adult acute lymphoblastic leukaemia)
- Minimising early and late toxicity of treatment

All patients who have either suspected or confirmed acute leukaemia should be referred for specialist advice, assessment, and treatment. Where a patient is referred to and the type of treatment given will depend on the patient's age and condition. Children and young adults should always be treated in recognised specialist centres to maximise the chance of cure with minimal toxicity. On admission to a specialist unit the patient will need chemotherapy to treat the leukaemia and supportive care to ameliorate or correct the effects of the leukaemia and to facilitate treatment.

Supportive care

Supportive care includes regular transfusions of platelet concentrate for bleeding episodes or if the platelet count is <15-$20\times10^9/l$; infusions of fresh frozen plasma if the coagulation screen results are abnormal;

and packed red cell transfusions for anaemia, though these are contraindicated if the white cell count is extremely high.

In most patients a central venous catheter has to be inserted to facilitate blood product support, administration of chemotherapy and antibiotics, and frequent blood sampling.

Serious infection is a common cause of death in patients with acute leukaemia as bone marrow failure due to the leukaemia and to chemotherapy often results in profound neutropenia for two weeks or more. Patients should therefore be reverse-barrier nursed, and intravenous antimicrobial agents should be started as soon as there is a fever or other sign of infection.

Chemotherapy

The aim of chemotherapy for leukaemia is initially to induce a remission (<5% blasts in the bone marrow) and then to eradicate the residual leukaemic cell population by further courses of consolidation therapy. The drugs damage the capacity of the leukaemic cells to divide and replicate, and using cyclical combinations of three or more drugs increases the cytotoxic effect, improves the chance of remission after the initial "induction" period, and reduces the emergence of drug resistance. In Britain acute myeloid leukaemia is currently treated with four courses of intensive chemotherapy, each of which entails five to 10 days of chemotherapy and then a period of three to five weeks before the next course. During this interval the patient is severely myelosuppressed and needs inpatient blood product support and antimicrobial drugs. In acute myeloid leukaemia M3 the drug ATRA (all-trans-retinoic acid) has been used as an adjunct to chemotherapy as it causes differentiation of the malignant clone.

In acute lymphoblastic leukaemia the induction course is followed by two or more consolidation periods and by treatment directed at the central nervous system (see below), followed by long term maintenance or continuation treatment for up to two years. This has been shown to improve long term cure rates in acute lymphoblastic leukaemia, though not in acute myeloid leukaemia.

Treatment directed at central nervous system

Treatment directed at the central nervous system is necessary to treat or prevent leukaemic cells in the central nervous system. Such treatment is part of all treatment protocols in childhood leukaemia and adult acute lymphoblastic leukaemia but not in adults with acute myeloid leukaemia unless they have symptoms or blasts are present in the cerebrospinal fluid. Treatment directed at the central nervous system generally comprises regular intrathecal chemotherapy (usually methotrexate), high dose intravenous methotrexate, or cranial irradiation.

Bone marrow transplantation

Allogeneic bone marrow transplantation may be curative in poor risk acute lymphoblastic leukaemia, acute myeloid leukaemia in first remission, or in relapsed leukaemia in which a second remission has been achieved. Transplantation is not available to all patients, however, owing to lack of compatible donors. Bone marrow transplantation is discussed in a later article.

Adequate hydration and allopurinol are essential at the start of treatment to reduce the risk of hyperkalaemia, hyperuricaemia, and renal damage

Psychological and social support to patients and families of patients with leukaemia is important, and specialist centres have networks to provide this

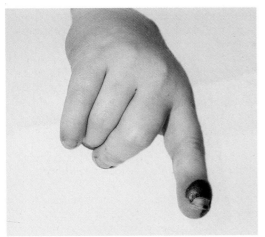

Figure 6.6 Pseudomonas infection of skin and nail bed in patient having treatment for acute myeloid leukaemia.

Ongoing Medical Research Council clinical trials

- Acute lymphoblastic leukaemia in both children and adults
- Relapsed acute lymphoblastic leukaemia in children
- Acute myeloid leukaemia in patients aged <60 years
- Acute myeloid leukaemia in patients aged >55 years

Survival with acute leukaemia

Type	At five years
Childhood acute lymphoblastic leukaemia	65-75%
Adult acute lymphoblastic leukaemia	20-35%
Acute myeloid leukaemia, aged <55 years	40-60%
Acute myeloid leukaemia, aged >55 years	20%

Poor prognosis in acute leukaemia

Factors	Acute lymphoblastic leukaemia	Acute myeloid leukaemia
Age	<1 Year or >10 years	>60 Years
Sex	Male	Male or female
Presenting white blood cells	>50 × 10⁹/l	>50 × 10⁹/l
Central nervous system disease	Presence of blasts in cerebrospinal fluid at presentation	Presence of blasts in cerebrospinal fluid at presentation (rare)
Remission problems	Failure to remit after first induction treatment	>20% Blasts in bone marrow after first course of treatment
Cytogenetics	Philadelphia positive—that is, t(9;22)—or t(4;11) acute lymphoblastic leukaemia	Deletions or monosomy of chromosome 5 or 7 or complex chromosomal abnormalities

Toxicity of therapy

Late effects of treatment for acute leukaemia

Cardiac—Arrhythmias, cardiomyopathy
Pulmonary—Fibrosis
Endocrine—Growth delay, hypothyroidism, gonadal
  dysfunction or failure, infertility
Renal—Reduced glomerular filtration rate
Psychological—Intellectual dysfunction, long term
  anxiety about relapse
Second malignancy—Secondary leukaemias or solid
  tumours
Cataracts

Early side effects

Most chemotherapeutic agents have pronounced side effects, such as nausea and vomiting, mucositis, hair loss, neuropathy, and renal and hepatic dysfunction. Many also cause myelosuppression, resulting in profound neutropenia for two or more weeks. Recurrent febrile neutropenic episodes require prompt and intensive antibiotics, and many patients also develop fungal infection requiring treatment with systemic antifungal drugs.

Late effects

All treatments for acute leukaemia can result in long term side effects that may bring appreciable morbidity—particularly in children—or even lead to death. All patients therefore need to be followed up for at least 10 years. In particular, the long term problems with growth and endocrine function in children need expert attention.

The interphase fluorescence in situ hybridisation was provided by Brian Reeves and Helen Kempski, department of haematology, Great Ormond Street Hospital for Children NHS Trust, London.

7 PLATELET DISORDERS

R J Liesner, S J Machin

Platelets are produced predominantly by bone marrow megakaryocytes as a result of budding of the cytoplasmic membrane. Megakaryocytes are derived from the haemopoietic stem cell, which is stimulated to differentiate to mature megakaryocytes under the influence of various cytokines, including thrombopoietin.

Once released from the bone marrow, young platelets are trapped in the spleen for 36 hours before entering the circulation, where they have a primary haemostatic role.

> The life span of a platelet is 7-10 days, and the normal count for all ages is $150-450\times10^9/l$

Normal haemostasis

The platelet membrane has integral glycoproteins essential in the initial events of adhesion and aggregation, leading to formation of the platelet plug during haemostasis.

Glycoprotein receptors react with aggregating agents such as collagen on the damaged endothelial surface (for example, blood vessels), fibrinogen, and von Willebrand's factor to facilitate platelet-platelet and platelet-endothelial cell adhesion. Storage organelles within the platelet include the "dense" granules, which contain nucleotides, calcium, and serotonin, and α granules containing fibrinogen, von Willebrand's factor, platelet derived growth factor, and many other clotting factors. After adhesion, platelets are stimulated to release the contents of their granules essential for platelet aggregation. Platelets also provide an extensive phospholipid surface for the interaction and activation of clotting factors in the coagulation cascade.

Congenital abnormalities

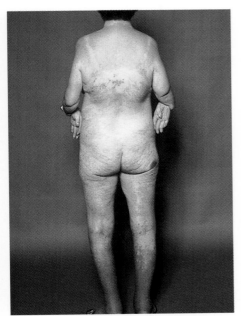

Figure 7.1 Amegakaryocytic thrombocytopenia with absent radii (TAR syndrome).

Congenital abnormalities can be disorders of platelet production or platelet function. All are very rare.

Fanconi's anaemia is an autosomal recessive preleukaemic condition that often presents as thrombocytopenia with skeletal or genitourinary abnormalities. The cardinal feature is abnormal chromosomal fragility. The condition can be cured only with bone marrow transplantation.

Amegakaryocytic thrombocytopenia presents with severe neonatal thrombocytopenia (platelet count $<2\times10^9/l$), though this often corrects itself after the first year of life. Infants with coexistent absent radii have the thrombocytopenia-absent radii (TAR) syndrome; they may also have the coexistent congenital cardiac defects.

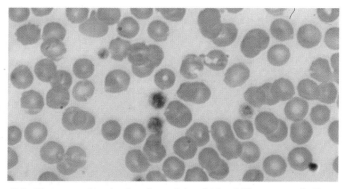

Figure 7.2 Giant granular platelets in peripheral blood film as seen in Bernard-Soulier syndrome or May-Hegglin anomaly.

> Diseases of the platelet storage pool are deficiencies in either the α or dense granules causing poor secondary platelet aggregation

The Wiskott-Aldrich syndrome is an X linked disorder with a triad of thrombocytopenia, eczema, and immunodeficiency. The platelet count is usually $20\text{-}100 \times 10^9/l$ and the platelets are functionally abnormal. Like Fanconi's anaemia, this condition can be cured only with bone marrow transplantation.

May-Hegglin anomaly and variants of Alport's syndrome are both characterised by giant platelets. The former is a benign condition, but the latter is associated with progressive hereditary nephritis and deafness.

Glanzmann's thrombasthenia, the Bernard-Soulier syndrome, and platelet-type von Willebrand's disease are characterised by absence or abnormalities of the glycoproteins in the platelet membrane, resulting in defective platelet adhesion and aggregation.

Acquired abnormalities

Acquired disorders of reduced platelet production*

- Drug induced
- Leukaemia
- Metastatic tumour
- Aplastic anaemia
- Myelodysplasia
- Cytotoxic drugs
- Radiotherapy
- Associated with infection
- Megaloblastic anaemia

* Due to bone marrow failure or replacement

Disorders with increased platelet consumption

- Disorders with immune mechanism
  Autoimmune—idiopathic thrombocytopenic purpura
  Alloimmune—post transfusion purpura, neonatal alloimmune thrombocytopenia
  Infection-associated—infectious mononucleosis, HIV, malaria
  Drug-induced—heparin, penicillin, quinine, sulphonamides, rifampicin
- Thrombotic thrombocytopenic purpura/haemolytic uraemic syndrome
- Hypersplenism and splenomegaly
- Disseminated intravascular coagulation
- Massive transfusion

Decreased production of platelets due to suppression or failure of the bone marrow is the commonest cause of thrombocytopenia. In aplastic anaemia, leukaemia, and marrow infiltration and after chemotherapy thrombocytopenia is usually associated with a failure of red and white cell production but may be an isolated finding secondary to drug toxicity (penicillamine, co-trimoxazole), alcohol, malaria, or viral infection (HIV, infectious mononucleosis). Viral infection is the most common cause of mild transient thrombocytopenia.

Increased platelet consumption may be due to immune or non-immune mechanisms. Idiopathic thrombocytopenic purpura is a relatively common disorder and the most frequent cause of isolated thrombocytopenia without anaemia or neutropenia. In adults it often presents insidiously, most frequently in women aged 15-50 years, and can be associated with other autoimmune diseases, in particular systemic lupus erythematosus or the primary antiphospholipid (lupus) syndrome. In children the onset is more acute and often follows a viral infection. The autoantibody produced is usually IgG, directed against antigens on the platelet membrane. Antibody-coated platelets are removed by the reticuloendothelial system, reducing the life span of the platelet to a few hours. The platelet count may vary from $<5 \times 10^9/l$ to near normal. The severity of bleeding is less than that seen with comparable degrees of thrombocytopenia in bone marrow failure due to the predominance of young, functionally superior platelets.

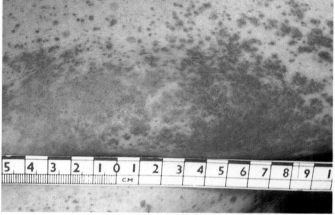

Figure 7.3 Spontaneous skin purpura in severe immune thrombocytopenia.

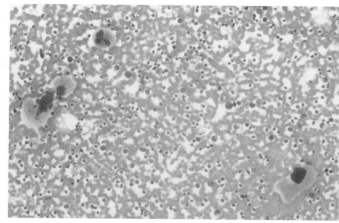

Figure 7.4 Bone marrow aspirate showing increased megakaryocytes in immune thrombocytopenia.

Post-transfusion purpura

- This is an acquired abnormality
- It is a rare complication of blood transfusion presenting with severe thrombocytopenia 7-10 days after the transfusion
- Patients are usually multiparous women who are negative for the human platelet antigen 1a
- Antibodies to this antigen develop that are somehow responsible for the immune destruction of the patient's own platelets

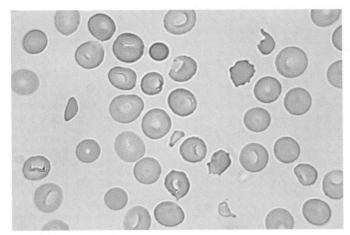

Figure 7.5 Red cell fragmentation in patient who presented with confusion and lethargy in whom thrombotic thrombocytopenic purpura was diagnosed. She responded well to large volume plasma exchange for one week.

Causes of acquired platelet dysfunction

- Aspirin and non-steroidal anti-inflammatory agents
- Penicillins and cephalosporins
- Uraemia
- Alcohol
- Liver disease
- Myeloproliferative disorders
- Myeloma
- Cardiopulmonary bypass
- Fish oils

Thrombocytosis

- Essential (primary) thrombocytosis
- Reactive (secondary) thrombocytosis
  - Infection
  - Malignant disease
  - Acute and chronic inflammatory diseases
  - Pregnancy
  - After splenectomy
  - Iron deficiency
  - Haemorrhage

Neonatal alloimmune thrombocytopenia is similar to haemolytic disease of newborn infants except that the antigenic stimulus comes from platelet specific antigens rather than red cell antigens. In 80% of cases the antigen is human platelet antigen 1a, and mothers negative for this antigen form antibodies when sensitised by a fetus positive for the antigen. Fetal platelet destruction results from transplacental passage of these antibodies, and severe bleeding including intracranial haemorrhage can occur in utero. Firstborn infants are frequently affected, and successive pregnancies are equally or more affected.

Heparin induced thrombocytopenia occurs during heparin treatment in up to 5% of patients. It may become manifest when arterial or venous thrombosis occurs during a fall in the platelet count and is thought to be due to the formation of antibodies to heparin that are bound to platelet factor 4, a platelet granule protein. The immune complexes activate platelets and endothelial cells, resulting in thrombocytopenia and thrombosis coexisting. Heparin induced thrombocytopenia carries an appreciable mortality risk if diagnosis is delayed.

Thrombotic thrombocytopenic purpura and the similar haemolytic uraemic syndrome cause fever, fluctuating neurological signs, renal impairment, and microvascular haemolysis, which results in thrombocytopenia. Red cell fragmentation on the blood film, a reticulocytosis, and the demonstration of an abnormal pattern of von Willebrand's multimers make the diagnosis highly likely.

Disseminated intravascular coagulation usually occurs in critically ill patients as a result of catastrophic activation of the coagulation pathway, often due to sepsis. Widespread platelet aggregation occurs, causing thrombocytopenia.

Massive splenomegaly—The spleen normally pools about a third of the platelet mass, but in massive splenomegaly the proportion can rise to 90%, resulting in apparent thrombocytopenia.

Aspirin and non-steroidal anti-inflammatory agents are the most common cause of acquired platelet dysfunction, and for this reason aspirin is now widely used therapeutically as an antiplatelet drug. It acts by irreversibly inhibiting cyclo-oxygenase activity in the platelet, resulting in impairment of the granule release reaction and defective aggregation. The effects of a single dose of aspirin last for the lifetime of the platelet (7-10 days).

Bleeding in uraemic patients is most commonly from defects in platelet adhesion or aggregation, though thrombocytopenia, severe anaemia with packed cell volume <20%, or coagulation defects can also contribute.

Essential (primary) thrombocytosis and *reactive (secondary) thrombocytosis*—In these conditions the platelet count is raised above the upper limit of normal. A wide range of disorders may cause a raised platelet count ($>1000\times10^9$/l), but patients are normally asymptomatic. However, antiplatelet drugs can be useful to prevent thrombosis in high risk patients—for example, postoperatively.

History and examination of patients

Prolonged nose bleeds are more likely in children than in adults

Abnormal bleeding associated with thrombocytopenia or abnormal platelet function is characterised by spontaneous skin purpura and ecchymoses, mucous membrane bleeding, and protracted bleeding after trauma. Prolonged nose bleeds can occur, and menorrhagia or postpartum haemorrhage is common in women.

Rarely, subconjunctival, retinal, gastrointestinal, genitourinary, or intracranial bleeds may occur. In thrombocytopenic patients severe spontaneous bleeding is unusual with a platelet count of $\geqslant 30 \times 10^9/l$.

Investigations

The investigations in a suspected platelet disorder will depend on the presentation and history in each patient

If the bleeding is severe the patient may need urgent hospital referral for prompt evaluation, diagnosis, and treatment, which may entail blood product support. All patients should have a full blood count, blood film, coagulation, and biochemical screen and then further investigations depending on the results of these.

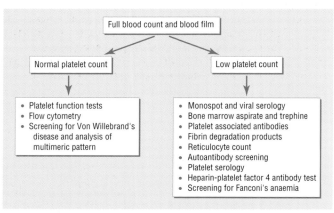

Figure 7.6 Investigation in a suspected platelet disorder.

Thrombocytopenia can be artefactual and due to platelet clumping or a blood clot in the sample, which should be excluded in all cases. The bleeding time (including the standard template technique) may or may not be prolonged in congenital or acquired platelet dysfunction, and therefore a normal bleeding time does not exclude these conditions. It is also not a good indicator of bleeding risk perioperatively.

Management

A neonate or small infant with bleeding must be referred for evaluation as the inherited bleeding disorders (eg haemophilia or von Willebrand's disease) and platelet disorders may present at a very young age

All serious bleeding due to a platelet disorder needs haematological assessment and treatment. Mild or trivial bleeding due to a transient postviral thrombocytopenia or aspirin needs no active treatment and can be managed in the community.

Treatment of platelet disorders

Congenital disorders
- Platelet transfusions (filtered)
- Desmopressin (DDAVP)
- Tranexamic acid

Acquired disorders
- Bone marrow failure—Platelet transfusions if platelet count is $<15 \times 10^9/l$
- Idiopathic thrombocytopenic purpura (adults)—Prednisolone, intravenous immunoglobulin, splenectomy
- Post-transfusion purpura—Intravenous immunoglobulin, plasma exchange
- Heparin induced thrombocytopenia—Anticoagulation, but without heparin
- Thrombotic thrombocytopenic purpura—Large volume plasma exchange, aspirin when platelets $>50 \times 10^9/l$
- Disseminated intravascular coagulation—Treatment of underlying cause, fresh frozen plasma, platelet transfusion
- Hypersplenism—Splenectomy if severe
- Platelet function disorders—Platelet transfusion, desmopressin (occasionally useful—for example, in uraemia)

Acquired disorders

In thrombocytopenia due to bone marrow failure or marrow infiltration—for example, leukaemia and cancer—prophylactic platelet transfusions are given to keep the platelet count above $15 \times 10^9/l$, though the threshold is higher in infected or bleeding patients or to cover invasive procedures.

In childhood idiopathic thrombocytopenic purpura spontaneous recovery is common, and treatment is given only in life threatening bleeding. In adults the condition rarely remits without treatment and is more likely to become chronic. Initial treatment is prednisolone 1 mg/kg daily (80% of cases remit) or intravenous immunoglobulin (0·4 g/kg for five days or 1 g/kg for two days), or both. In refractory patients splenectomy has a 60-70%

chance of long term remission, and azathioprine, danazol, vinca alkaloids, and high dose dexamethasone have all been tried with variable success.

Post-transfusion purpura may respond to intravenous immuno-globulin (at doses given above), or plasma exchange may be required. Platelet transfusions should be avoided.

Patients in whom heparin induced thrombocytopenia is suspected are often inpatients with ongoing thrombosis who may have complex medical problems. It is essential to withdraw heparin and treat thrombosis with anticoagulants, avoiding all forms of heparin. Warfarin, synthetic heparinoids, or ancrod can be used. Platelet transfusions are contraindicated in heparin induced thrombocytopenia and in thrombotic thrombocytopenic purpura. If the latter is suspected clinically and on the basis of laboratory tests, large volume plasma exchange should be started immediately and continued daily until substantial clinical improvement and all the results of haematological tests have normalised. Aspirin can be started once the platelet count is $> 50 \times 10^9/l$.

With disseminated intravascular coagulation it is essential to treat the underlying cause as well as to support depletion of clotting factors and platelets with blood products.

In pronounced bleeding or risk of bleeding due to the acquired disorders of platelet function platelets usually have to be transfused to provide normally functioning platelets, though desmopressin (DDAVP) and tranexamic acid can also be of value. Usually treatment may only be necessary to cover surgical procedures or major haemorrhage.

8 THE MYELODYSPLASTIC SYNDROMES

David G Oscier

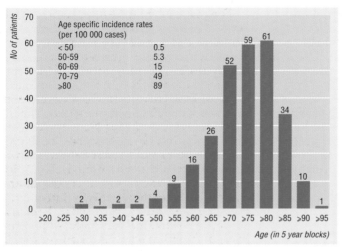

Age specific incidence rates (per 100 000 cases)

< 50	0.5
50-59	5.3
60-69	15
70-79	49
≥80	89

Figure 8.1 Age distribution and incidence rates per 100 000 population of patients presenting with myelodysplastic syndrome in Bournemouth,1981-90.

The term myelodysplastic syndromes was introduced in 1975 by a group of French, American, and British haematologists (FAB group) to describe a group of disorders with characteristic abnormalities of peripheral blood and bone marrow morphology and impaired bone marrow function, which tend to evolve into acute myeloid leukaemia. Although the myelodysplastic syndromes may occur at any age, they are predominantly diseases of elderly people.

Aetiology

Primary myelodysplastic syndrome describes those cases—the majority—in which the cause is unknown. Case-control studies have shown a modest correlation between the myelodysplastic syndromes and exposure to low doses of radiation and organic chemicals.

Therapy related myelodysplastic syndrome, sometimes called secondary myelodysplastic syndrome, describes cases that have arisen as a long term complication of cytotoxic chemotherapy. The risk is highest 4-10 years after treatment with alkylating agents, such as chlorambucil and cyclophosphamide.

Diagnosis

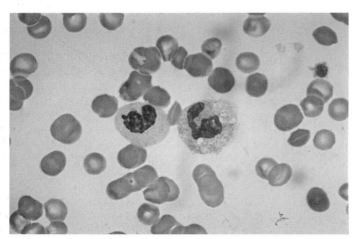

Figure 8.2 Blood film showing normal neutrophil (right) and dysplastic neutrophil with agranular cytoplasm and hypolobated nucleus.

Patients present with the features of bone marrow failure—namely, symptoms of anaemia, bacterial infections, and bleeding or bruising. Splenomegaly is present in about 10% of patients, particularly in chronic myelomonocytic leukaemia, one subtype of the myelodysplastic syndromes. Increasingly, myelodysplastic syndrome is an incidental finding in elderly patients whose routine blood count shows an unexplained anaemia, macrocytosis, neutropenia, monocytosis, or thrombocytopenia.

The myelodysplastic syndromes can be diagnosed only by a haematologist, primarily on the basis of characteristic full blood count indices, morphological abnormalities on the peripheral blood film, and characteristic bone marrow appearances. Although myelodys-

Morphological abnormalities in myelodysplastic syndrome

Lineage	Blood	Marrow
Erythroid	Oval macrocytes	Abnormal nuclear shape and chromatin pattern
	Basophilic stippling	Ring sideroblasts
Myeloid	Hypogranular neutrophils	
	Hypolobated neutrophil nuclei	
Megakaryocytic	Agranular platelets	Micromegakaryocytes
		Mononuclear megakaryocytes
		Megakaryocytes with separated nuclei

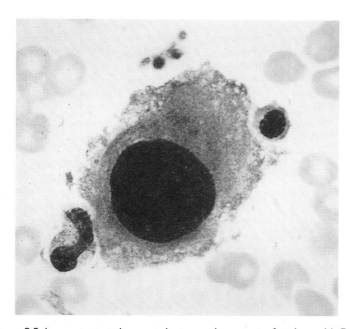

Figure 8.3 Large mononuclear megakaryocyte in marrow of patient with 5q⁻ syndrome.

plastic syndrome may sometimes be diagnosed on the basis of a blood film alone, a bone marrow aspirate and trephine are necessary to make a confident diagnosis and to assess the severity of the disease. Marrow examination can safely be omitted only in elderly, infirm patients with mild cytopenias who would not need treatment regardless of the marrow findings.

Diagnosis is frequently straightforward, particularly if morphological abnormalities are found in the three major lineages—erythroid (red cells), myeloid (granulocytes, including neutrophils), and megakaryocytic series (platelets)—in the clinical context of an elderly patient with a peripheral blood cytopenia. However, morphological dysplasia is not synonymous with myelodysplastic syndrome, and similar morphological abnormalities to those found in early myelodysplastic syndromes may be seen in vitamin B_{12} deficiency or folate deficiency, alcohol excess, after cytotoxic chemotherapy, HIV infection, and even in a minority of cells in the bone marrow of normal individuals. Problems also arise if morphological abnormalities are subtle, if they involve only one cell lineage, or if the staining of blood and marrow slides is suboptimal.

Chromosome analysis

Cytogenetic analysis of bone marrow should be performed whenever the diagnosis of myelodysplastic syndrome is suspected from the blood film. It is valuable both prognostically and when the morphological diagnosis is difficult. A clonal chromosome abnormality—that is, the same abnormality appearing in more than one cell—confirms the presence of a primary bone marrow disorder and excludes the reactive causes of dysplasia listed above. Chromosomal abnormalities are found in 30-50% of cases of primary myelodysplastic syndrome and in 80% of cases of therapy related myelodysplastic syndrome. Specific chromosomal abnormalities may be associated with particular clinical and haematological features. For example, loss of part of a long arm ("q") of chromosome 5 occurring as the only chromosomal abnormality (5q⁻ syndrome) is associated with macrocytic anaemia in elderly women and a low risk or transformation to acute myeloid leukaemia. Loss of the short arm ("p") of chromosome 17 is found in advanced disease and is associated with drug resistance and short survival.

Most of the chromosomal abnormalities in the myelodysplastic syndromes involve loss of genetic material, but the critical genes that are deleted are yet to be discovered. Disease progression, particularly evolution to acute leukaemia, is frequently accompanied by additional chromosomal abnormalities ("karyotypic evolution").

Chromosome abnormalities in myelodysplasia

Abnormality	Incidence(%)	
	Primary myelodysplastic syndrome	Therapy related myelodysplastic syndrome
Deletion of 5q	10-20	20
Monosomy 7	10-15	30-50
Trisomy 8	15	10
Loss of 17p	3	10

FAB classification

In 1982 the FAB group divided the myelodysplastic syndromes into five subgroups based on (*a*) the percentage of immature myeloid cells (blast cells) and ring sideroblasts (immature red cells with iron granules arranged in a ring around the nucleus) in the bone marrow and (*b*) the presence or absence of a raised peripheral blood monocyte count. This classification was rapidly adopted worldwide and is still widely used. Individual subgroups, however, should not be viewed as distinct disorders as patients may pass through several stages during the course of their disease. Although chronic myelomonocytic leukaemia shares the morphological abnormalities common to all the myelodysplastic syndromes, many patients have features such as leucocytosis and splenomegaly, which are more typical of a myeloproliferative disorder. Patients with more than 30% blasts in the bone marrow are considered to have acute leukaemia, but the distinction between myelodysplasia with more than 20% blasts and acute myeloid leukaemia in elderly people is blurred. Elderly people with acute myeloid leukaemia often have dysplastic morphology, similar chromosomal abnormalities, and a similar clinical course to patients with advanced myelodysplastic syndromes.

FAB classification of myelodysplastic syndrome

Category	Peripheral blood		Bone marrow
Refractory anaemia (RA)	<1% blasts	*and*	<5% blasts
Refractory anaemia with ring sideroblasts (RARS)	<1% blasts	*and*	<5% blasts, >15% ring sideroblasts
Refractory anaemia with excess blasts (RAEB)	<5% blasts	*and*	5-20% blasts
Refractory anaemia with excess blasts in transformation (RAEBt)	>5% blasts	*or*	21-30% blasts
Chronic myelomonocytic leukaemia (CMML)	$>1\times10^9/l$ Monocytes		

Natural course and prognosis

Median survival (months) of primary myelodysplastic syndrome according to FAB type

FAB type	Median survival	Range
All cases	20	7·4–28
Refractory anaemia	50	18–64
Refractory anaemia with ring sideroblasts	51	14–76
Refractory anaemia with excess blasts	13	7–21
Refractory anaemia with excess blasts in transformation	6	2·5–16
Chronic myelomonocytic leukaemia	18	4 to >60

The clinical course of the myelodysplastic syndromes is extremely variable even among patients of the same subgroup. About two thirds of patients die of marrow failure (of whom half undergo leukaemic transformation), and one third die of unrelated causes. The median survival of patients with myelodysplastic syndrome is 20 months and for all subtypes is shorter than that of age matched controls.

Although the FAB classification has prognostic significance, a more accurate prediction of survival can be achieved by using a scoring system that incorporates the presenting haemoglobin concentration, neutrophil and platelet counts, the percentage of blasts in the bone marrow, and chromosome abnormalities.

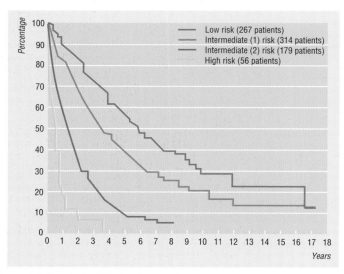

Figure 8.4 Survival of 816 patients who had received no treatment or only supportive care on the basis of the international scoring system.

International prognostic scoring system for myelodysplastic syndrome

Prognostic variable	Score*				
	0	0·5	1·0	1·5	2·0
Marrow blasts (%)	<5	5-10	–	11-20	21-30
Karyotype	Good†	Intermediate‡	Poor¶		
Cytopenias	0/1	2/3			

* 0=low risk, 0·5-1·0=intermediate risk 1,1·5-2·0=intermediate risk 2, ≥2·5=high risk.
† Normal karyotype or absent Y chromosome (−Y), deletion of long arm of chromosomes 5 or 20 (del(5q), del(20q)).
‡ Other abnormalities.
¶ Complex karyotypic abnormalities (≥3 abnormalities), or chromosome 7 anomalies.

Management decisions should not be based on blood and marrow samples taken during severe bacterial infections as infections can result in acute and reversible changes in the neutrophil and platelet counts and the percentage of marrow blasts.

Management

Treatment options in myelodysplasia

- Observation
- Supportive care
  Red cell or platelet transfusions, or both
  Antibiotics
  Haemopoietic growth factors
- Intensive chemotherapy
- Low dose chemotherapy
- Differentiating agents
- Bone marrow transplantation

The treatment of the myelodysplastic syndromes is generally unsatisfactory, which partially accounts for the variety of therapeutic options.

Before the most appropriate treatment can be determined, several factors must be taken into consideration. These include the patient's age and general fitness, the severity of the disease at presentation, prognostic factors, and whether the disease is stable or progressive. Consequently, whenever possible there should be a period of observation before a decision about long term treatment is made.

For most patients treatment is palliative, and the possibility of cure applies only to the minority of young patients suitable for an allogeneic bone marrow transplant. Sixty per cent of such patients without an increase in marrow blasts and 40% of patients with increased blasts will be free of disease five years after transplantation.

Low risk patients need observation only. For fit and well motivated patients under the age of 65-70 years with intermediate or poor risk disease, intensive chemotherapy currently offers the best possibility of improved quality and duration of life. Remission rates of 60% are achievable but rarely last beyond 18 months.

Low dose cytotoxic treatment with hydroxyurea or etoposide may reduce spleen size and improve the blood count in patients with intermediate and poor risk chronic myelomonocytic leukaemia, but the median survival remains poor at less than two years.

Drugs that could induce the differentiation of immature into mature myeloid cells without causing bone marrow toxicity would be highly prized in the treatment of the myelodysplastic syndromes. Low dose cytosine arabinoside and analogues of vitamin D3 and retinoic acid have differentiating activity in vitro but so far have been disappointing in clinical use.

The cornerstone of the treatment of the myelodysplastic syndromes remains the judicious use of red cell and platelet transfusions and antibiotics for most elderly patients with symptomatic disease. Iron chelation therapy should be considered for patients who need red cell transfusion long term. Recombinant growth factors can improve the neutrophil count in over 90% of patients (granulocyte-colony stimulating factor or granulocyte-macrophage colony stimulating factor) and the haemoglobin concentration in 20-40% of patients (erythropoietin with or without either

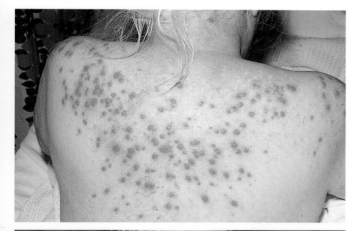
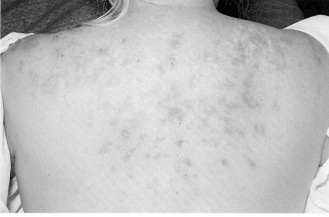

Figure 8.5 70 Year old woman with refractory anaemia with excess blasts in transformation showing improvement in leukaemic skin deposits after course of low dose cytosine arabinoside.

of these colony stimulating factors). Intermittent administration of either of these colony stimulating factors may be considered in patients with severe neutropenia and recurrent infections. Growth factors are expensive, however, and least effective in patients with advanced disease and severe cytopenias—those who most require treatment.

The histogram showing age distribution and incidence rates for myelodysplastic syndrome is adapted with permission from the *British Journal of Haematology* (Williamson PJ, Kruger AR, Reynolds PJ, Hamblin TJ, Oscier DG. Establishing the incidence of myelodysplastic syndrome. 1994;87:743-5). The illustration of the mononuclear megakaryocyte is reproduced with permission from *Leukaemia Diagnosis: A Guide to the FAB Classification* (Bain B, London: Mosby International, 1993).

Further reading

- Mufti GJ, Galton DAG. *The myelodysplastic syndromes*. Edinburgh: Churchill Livingstone, 1992.
- Koeffler HP, ed. *Seminars in hematology. The myelodysplastic syndromes. Parts I and II.* Philadelphia:Saunders, 1996.

9 MULTIPLE MYELOMA AND RELATED CONDITIONS

Charles R J Singer

Charles R J Singer

Conditions associated with M proteins

Stable production
- Monoclonal gammopathy of undetermined significance
- Smouldering multiple myeloma

Progressive production
- Multiple myeloma (IgG, IgA, free light chains, IgD, IgE)
- Plasma cell leukaemia
- Solitary plasmacytoma of bone
- Extramedullary plasmacytoma
- Waldenström's macroglobulinaemia (IgM)
- Chronic lymphocytic leukaemia
- Malignant lymphoma
- Primary amyloidosis
- Heavy chain disease

Multiple myeloma

Clinical features of myeloma

Common
- Bone pain and pathological fractures
- Anaemia and bone marrow failure
- Infection due to immune paresis and neutropenia
- Renal impairment

Less common
- Acute hypercalcaemia
- Symptomatic hyperviscosity
- Neuropathy
- Amyloidosis
- Coagulopathy

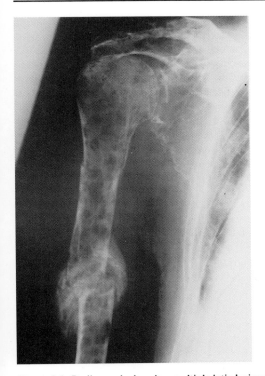

Figure 9.1 Radiograph showing multiple lytic lesions and pathological fractures of humerus.

The plasma cell dyscrasias represent a heterogeneous group of conditions characterised by disordered proliferation of monoclonal plasma cells, most of which produce monoclonal immunoglobulin (M protein or paraprotein) in the serum or urine. The clinical phenotype is determined by the rate of accumulation and the biological properties of the abnormal cells and the monoclonal protein.

The incidence of myeloma is about 4 per 100 000 in Britain. It is more than twice as high in African Americans as in white Americans and Europeans, although it is much lower among Chinese and Japanese Asians. Myeloma is extremely rare in people aged under 40 years, but its incidence increases to over 30 per 100 000 in those aged over 80. The median age at diagnosis is 69 years, with slight male predominance.

Pathogenesis and clinical features

Myeloma is due to unregulated, progressive proliferation of neoplastic monoclonal plasma cells that accumulate in the marrow, leading to anaemia and marrow failure. The cell of origin is probably a memory B lymphocyte, and neoplastic cells home to the bone marrow, where the environment rich in interleukin 6 stimulates proliferation of plasma cells.

Myeloma cells produce and secrete a monoclonal protein, usually intact immunoglobulin. IgG paraprotein is present in 60% of cases and IgA in 20-25%, and in 15-20% of cases free immunoglobulin light chains alone are produced. Myelomas whose cells secrete IgD, two clonal proteins, IgM, or no protein are rare. Free light chains are detectable in urine as Bence Jones protein.

Accumulation of M protein may lead to hyperviscosity (especially IgA and IgM polymers) or deposition of the protein in renal tubules, resulting in renal failure. Production of normal immunoglobulin is often depressed (immune paresis) and contributes to the patient's susceptibility to infection.

Bone destruction is characteristic, and the associated bone pain a major cause of morbidity in myeloma. Myeloma is associated with abnormal bone remodelling due to increased osteoclastic bone resorption and inhibition of osteoblastic bone formation. This results in pronounced bone loss and the characteristic osteolytic lesions predisposing to pathological fractures. Widespread bone destruction may lead to hypercalcaemia, resulting in a vicious cycle of dehydration, worsening hypercalcaemia, and renal failure.

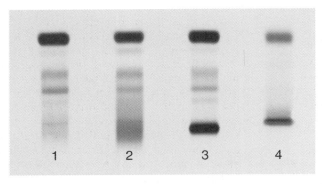

Figure 9.2 Protein electrophoresis strip showing (1) normal plasma, (2) polyclonal hypergammaglobulinaemia, (3) serum M protein, and (4) urine M protein (Bence Jones proteinuria) and albuminuria.

The most common presenting complaint is bone pain, commonly affecting the back. Symptoms of anaemia, renal failure, or infection are also frequent. Less common are symptoms of hyperviscosity (impaired central nervous system, impaired vision, purpura, and haemorrhage), acute hypercalcaemia, spinal cord compression, neuropathy, or amyloidosis. About 20% of patients are asymptomatic, and diagnosis results from routine investigations.

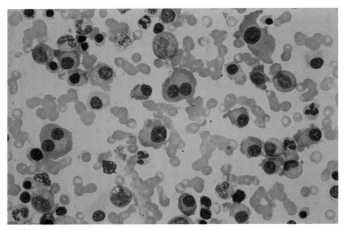

Figure 9.3 Bone marrow aspirate showing infiltrate of abnormal plasma cells (medium power).

Investigations and diagnosis

Myeloma should be suspected in anyone aged over 40 years with unexplained bone pain or fracture, osteoporosis, osteolytic lesions, lethargy, anaemia, red cell rouleaux, raised erythrocyte sedimentation rate or plasma viscosity, hypercalcaemia, renal dysfunction, proteinuria, or recurrent infection. It is characterised by the classic triad of infiltration of the bone marrow by plasma cells, lytic bone lesions on skeletal radiology, and the presence of M protein in the serum or urine, or in both.

History and examination should be followed by a full blood count and film; erythrocyte sedimentation rate or plasma viscosity; urea and creatinine concentrations; calcium, phosphate, and alkaline phosphatase concentrations; uric acid concentration; serum protein electrophoresis; measurement of serum immunoglobulins; routine urine analysis; urine electrophoresis for Bence Jones protein; skeletal survey; and bone marrow aspirate and biopsy.

Normochromic normocytic anaemia is often present; neutropenia and thrombocytopenia suggest advanced disease. Rouleaux are usually seen in the blood film, and plasma cells may also be present in about 5% of cases. The erythrocyte sedimentation rate and plasma viscosity are often noticeably increased but are normal in 10% of cases. The serum calcium concentration is increased in up to 20% of cases, with normal alkaline phosphatase concentration. Raised urea and creatinine concentrations occur in 20% of cases. Low serum albumin concentration reflects advanced disease. Skeletal radiology shows lytic lesions or generalised bone rarefaction in 80% of cases. Bone scans are typically negative in multiple myeloma despite extensive bone damage.

The most important differential diagnosis is between multiple myeloma and monoclonal gammopathy of undetermined significance (for which no treatment is indicated). No single test differentiates the two conditions reliably. A serum IgG concentration > 30 g/l or IgA concentration > 20 g/l suggests a diagnosis of myeloma rather than monoclonal gammopathy of undetermined significance. Some patients have "smouldering multiple myeloma," in which M protein and bone marrow criteria exist for the diagnosis of myeloma, but anaemia, renal impairment, and skeletal lesions do not develop and the M protein and plasma cells remain stable. Here too a "watch and wait" policy is appropriate.

Minimal diagnostic criteria for myeloma

- > 10% Plasma cells in bone marrow or plasmacytoma on biopsy
- Clinical features of myeloma
- Plus at least one of:
    Serum M band (IgG > 30 g/l; IgA > 20 g/l)
    Urine M band (Bence Jones proteinuria)
    Osteolytic lesions on skeletal survey

If myeloma is suspected a urine sample should always be analysed for Bence Jones proteinuria as solitary free light chains are commonly undetected by routine serum electrophoresis

Laboratory findings at diagnosis (proportion of cases)

• Normochromic normocytic anaemia	60%
• Increased erythrocyte sedimentation rate or plasma viscosity	90%
• Serum M protein	80%
• Urine M protein only	20%
• Raised serum calcium concentration	20%
• Raised serum creatinine concentration	25%
• Proteinuria	70%

Management and clinical course

Without treatment a patient with multiple myeloma is likely to experience progressive bone damage, anaemia, and renal failure.

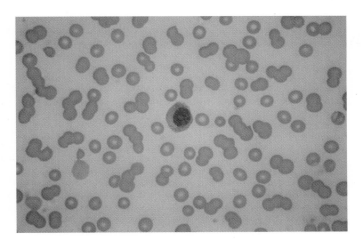

Figure 9.4 Blood film rouleaux and abnormal plasma cells (medium power).

Features of poor prognosis at diagnosis

- Low haemoglobin concentration (<85 g/l)
- Hypercalcaemia
- Advanced lytic bone lesions
- High M protein production rates (IgG >70 g/l; IgA >50 g/l; Bence Jones protein >12 g/24h)
- Abnormal renal function
- High plasma cell proliferative index
- Low serum albumin concentration (<30 g/l)
- High β2-microglobulin concentration (>6 mg/ml)

Treatment considerations in myeloma

- Analgesia
- Rehydration
- Treatment of any hypercalcaemia
- Treatment of any renal impairment
- Treatment of any infection
- Local radiotherapy if required
- Chemotherapy
- Prevention of further bone damage

Infection is the most common cause of death. Initial treatment should consist of (a) adequate analgesia—opiates often, and local radiotherapy to fractures or osteolytic lesions may have dramatic benefit; (b) rehydration—patients are often dehydrated at presentation, even without hypercalcaemia or renal impairment; (c) management of hypercalcaemia if present—rehydration, diuresis, and if necessary bisphosphonate therapy; (d) management of renal impairment—rehydration and treatment of any hypercalcaemia often have a pronounced effect on abnormal serum chemistry in myeloma, though in some patients only careful chemotherapy or dialysis, or both, is effective; (e) treatment of any infection—most infections at diagnosis are bacterial and respiratory and respond to broad spectrum antibiotics, though later in the disease antifungal treatment may be necessary; and (f) chemotherapy.

Oral melphalan and prednisolone administered in four day pulses at intervals of four to six weeks produces >50% reduction in the M protein concentration in 50% of patients. The treatment is well tolerated, but complete responses are rare. The median survival is about three years. During the plateau phase clinical and laboratory results should be reviewed at regular intervals to identify progression at the earliest opportunity. Further treatment (with melphalan) may then induce another plateau phase.

Combination intravenous chemotherapeutic regimens may produce higher response rates (up to 70%) and may improve survival. Combination regimens may be more effective in younger patients with high tumour loads, though they may be more toxic in elderly patients.

High dose melphalan and autologous stem cell transplantation after initial treatment produces a complete response in up to 75% of patients and prolongs survival but is not curative. It is applicable only to younger patients.

Allogeneic bone marrow transplantation may cure the condition but with considerable treatment related morbidity and mortality.

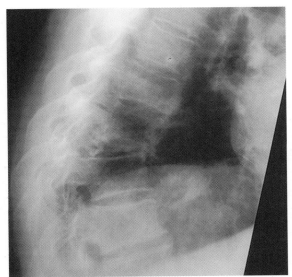

Figure 9.5 Bone pain from mechanical effects of myeloma damage (as in spine shown here) often necessitates long term treatment with strong analgesia despite response to chemotherapy.

Plateau phase

In most patients a stable partial response is achieved in which at least a 50% reduction in the M protein has occurred but chemotherapy fails to produce a further fall over a three month period. A plateau phase may occur in which cessation of chemotherapy may not be followed by a rise in the M band or further signs of progression for many months. Maintenance interferon alfa may prolong the plateau phase by six to 12 months, but little evidence exists of an effect on survival. Bisphosphonate treatment reduces the rate of further bone damage and may have an additive analgesic effect in patients with pre-existing damage and a survival benefit.

Options for initial chemotherapy in myeloma

- Melphalan with or without prednisolone
- Infusional chemotherapy—vincristine and adriamycin infusion plus either dexamethasone or methylprednisolone
- Combination therapy—for example, adriamycin, carmustine, cyclophosphamide, and melphalan
- Weekly cyclophosphamide ("C weekly")

Disease progression

With regular follow up, serological detection of disease will allow chemotherapy to be restarted before new bone damage develops, and in many patients several separate periods of plateau phase may be re-induced by chemotherapy. Inevitably myeloma becomes resistant to melphalan; oral dexamethasone may achieve further responses, and oral low dose cyclophosphamide daily is often effective palliative treatment in combination with local radiotherapy to sites of bone pain.

Conditions related to multiple myeloma

Diagnostic criteria for monoclonal gammopathy of undetermined significance

- No unexplained symptoms suggestive of myeloma
- Serum M protein concentration < 30 g/l
- < 5% Plasma cells in bone marrow
- Little or no M protein in urine
- No bone lesions
- No anaemia, hypercalcaemia, or renal impairment
- M protein concentration and other results stable on prolonged observation

> No treatment for monoclonal gammopathy of undetermined significance is indicated, but follow up is necessary

Plasma cell leukaemia

- May be diagnosed when blood plasma cells exceed $2 \cdot 0 \times 10^9$/l
- May occur as a terminal stage in advanced multiple myeloma or as aggressive disease at diagnosis in under 5% of cases
- Bone involvement is often minimal, and the M protein concentration is often low
- Results of treatment are poor, but intensive treatment can induce responses and prolong survival

Clinical and laboratory features of Waldenström's macroglobulinaemia

- Fatigue and weight loss
- Anaemia
- Hyperviscosity syndrome (may cause chronic oral or nasal bleeding, visual upset, headache, vertigo, hearing loss, ataxia, somnolence, and coma)
- Retinal haemorrhages
- Venous congestion (sausage formation) in retinal veins
- Recurrent infection
- Lymphadenopathy
- Hepatosplenomegaly
- Raised erythrocyte sedimentation rate
- High serum monoclonal IgM concentration
- Lymphoplasmacytoid bone marrow infiltrate

Further reading

- Kyle RA. Diagnostic criteria of multiple myeloma. *Hematol Oncol Clin North Am* 1992;6:347-58.
- Kyle RA. Monoclonal gammopathy of undetermined significance. *Baillières Clin Haematol* 1995;8:761-81.
- Bergsagel DE. The role of chemotherapy in the treatment of multiple myeloma. *Baillières Clin Haematol* 1995;8:783-94.

Monoclonal gammopathy of undetermined significance

Monoclonal gammopathy of undetermined significance is defined by the presence of an M protein in a patient without multiple myeloma, Waldenström's macroglobulinaemia, amyloidosis, lymphoma, or other related disease. The prevalence of monoclonal gammopathy of undetermined significance is about 20 times greater than that of multiple myeloma, and the incidence increases with age (1% at over 50 years; 3% at over 70).

Multiple myeloma, macroglobulinaemia, amyloidosis, or lymphoma ultimately develops in 26% of patients with monoclonal gammopathy of undetermined significance, with an actuarial rate of 16% at 10 years.

Solitary plasmacytoma

About 5% of patients have a single bone lesion at diagnosis with no evidence of disseminated bone marrow involvement. Generally M protein is absent (up to 70% of cases) or present in low concentration. Plasmacytoma may be cured by local radiotherapy. Patients with solitary plasmacytoma should be monitored for evidence of myeloma, which develops in most cases. Further plasmacytomas may develop, and magnetic resonance imaging may show bone lesions undetectable by conventional radiology. Median survival is over 10 years.

Waldenström's macroglobulinaemia

This condition is the result of proliferation of lymphocytes and plasma cells which produce monoclonal IgM. The median age at presentation is 63 years, and over 60% of patients are male. Many of the clinical features are the result of hyperviscosity due to the raised IgM concentration.

Weakness, fatigue, and bleeding are the most common presenting complaints, followed by visual upset, weight loss, recurrent infections, dyspnoea, heart failure, and neurological symptoms. Bone pain is rare.

The erythrocyte sedimentation rate is greatly raised, and when the plasma viscosity exceeds 4 cP most patients have symptoms of hyperviscosity. Serum protein immunoelectrophoresis shows an IgM paraprotein concentration often exceeding 30 g/l. Monoclonal light chains may be present in the urine. Trephine biopsy often shows extensive infiltration with plasmacytoid lymphocytes.

Symptomatic hyperviscosity is corrected by plasmapheresis. Chlorambucil with or without prednisolone for one week every four to six weeks frequently reduces bone marrow infiltration, the IgM concentration, and plasma viscosity. Median survival is about five years.

Other related conditions

Chronic lymphocytic leukaemia and diffuse low grade non-Hodgkin's lymphoma may be associated with low serum concentrations of monoclonal IgG or IgM. This finding has no prognostic importance for patients with these diseases. Primary amyloidosis is associated with an M protein in 85% of cases. The "heavy chain diseases" are rare lymphoproliferative disorders in which the abnormal cells excrete only parts of immunoglobulin heavy chains (γ, α, or μ).

The slide of the protein electrophoresis strip was provided by Mr D Costello.

10 BLEEDING DISORDERS, THROMBOSIS, AND ANTICOAGULATION

K K Hampton, F E Preston

Blood within the vascular tree remains fluid throughout life, but if a blood vessel is damaged, blood will clot in a rapid localised response. Failure of clotting leads to bleeding disorders; thrombosis is inappropriate clotting within blood vessels. The haemostatic system is complex, and many congenital and acquired conditions can disturb its correct functioning.

Bleeding disorders

History in bleeding disorders

- Abnormal bruising
- Abnormal bleeding from cuts and abrasions
- Nose bleeds
- Menorrhagia
- Haemarthrosis
- Bleeding after dental extraction
- Bleeding during childbirth
- Bleeding during surgery
- Previous anaemia and transfusions
- Drug history
- Family history

Persistent menorrhagia sufficient to cause iron deficiency anaemia may indicate a bleeding disorder if no structural uterine abnormality is present

---

Screening tests for bleeding disorders

Test	Abnormality detected
Blood count and film	Anaemia, leukaemia, disseminated intravascular coagulation
Platelet count	Thrombocytopenia
Activated partial thromboplastin time	Deficiency of all coagulation factors except VII, especially factors VIII and IX; heparin
Prothrombin time	Deficiency of factors I, II, V, VII, and X; warfarin
Thrombin time or fibrinogen	Hypofibrinogenaemia or dysfibrinogenaemia; heparin; fibrin degradation products
Bleeding time	Test of platelet-vessel wall interaction

Patients who have unexplained abnormalities on screening investigations should be referred for special management

---

History

Personal and family history is as important as laboratory investigation in assessing bleeding disorders. Easy bruising, nose bleeds (especially in children), and menorrhagia are common and do not necessarily signify a haemostatic defect unless they are persistent and severe. Small bruises on the limbs in response to minor trauma and simple easy bruising are especially common in elderly people and those receiving long term corticosteroids.

Large bruises after minimal trauma and on the trunk may indicate an important haemostatic defect. Abnormally prolonged bleeding from minor cuts and scratches and delayed recurrence of bleeding are also important, as is gum bleeding if there is no gingival disease and if it is unrelated to the trauma of brushing. Repeated nose bleeds lasting more than 10 minutes despite compression suggest a local cause or an underlying bleeding disorder.

The haemostatic response to previous haemostatic challenges is informative, especially in mild conditions when spontaneous bleeding is rare. A history of excessive bleeding or recurrence of bleeding after dental extractions, circumcision, tonsillectomy, other previous surgical operations, and childbirth should be sought, as should a history of unexplained anaemia, gastrointestinal bleeding without the demonstration of a cause, and previous blood transfusion.

A drug history should be taken to assess intake of aspirins and nonsteroidal anti-inflammatory drugs, and appropriate questioning will suggest causes for acquired haemostatic disorders, such as excessive alcohol intake, liver disease, or renal disease.

An inherited bleeding condition will result in a family history of the condition and suggest a pattern of inheritance—for example, autosomal dominant inheritance (both sexes affected) or X linked inheritance (only males affected).

In severe coagulation factor deficiency, such as haemophilia A or B, bleeding occurs primarily into muscles and joints, whereas in platelet disorders and von Willebrand's disease bleeding tends to be mucocutaneous—for example, nose bleeds, menorrhagia, and gum and gastrointestinal bleeding.

Laboratory investigation

The vast majority of important bleeding disorders can be excluded if the findings are all normal for blood and platelet counts; blood film; prothrombin time; activated partial thromboplastin time; fibrinogen or thrombin time; and bleeding time. These tests will reveal quantitative

Clinical features of coagulation factor deficiency and platelet type/von Willebrand's disease

	Coagulation defect	Platelet/von Willebrand's disease
Bruises	Large, on body and limbs	Small
Bleeding from cuts	Not severe	Profuse
Nose bleeds	Not common	Common, often prolonged and severe
Gastrointestinal bleeding	Uncommon, no underlying lesion	Common
Haemarthrosis	Common in severe haemophilia	Very uncommon
Haematuria	Common	Rare
Bleeding after dental extraction and surgery	Delayed 12-24 hours after haemostatic challenge	From time of challenge

Clinical severity of haemophilia A and B

Factor value*	Bleeding tendency
<0·02	Severe—frequent spontaneous bleeding into joints, muscles, and internal organs
0·02-0·05	Moderate—some "spontaneous" bleeds, bleeding after minor trauma
>0·05	Mild—bleeding only after significant trauma or surgery

* Normal value of factors VIII and IX is 0.5-1.5

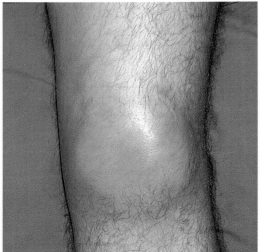

Figure 10.1 Acute haemarthrosis of knee joint.

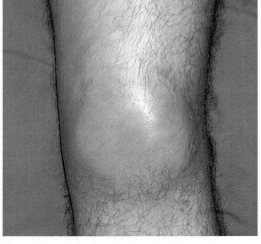

Figure 10.2 Pathological bruising in von Willebrand's disease.

Acquired bleeding disorders

Disease	Pathophysiology
Liver disease and cirrhosis	Decreased synthesis of coagulation factors, thrombocytopenia
Gastrointestinal malabsorption	Vitamin K deficiency
Shock/sepsis/malignancy	Disseminated intravascular coagulation, increased consumption of coagulation factors and platelets
Renal disease	Acquired platelet dysfunction
Lymphoproliferative disorders/spontaneous	Acquired autoantibodies to specific coagulation factors (inhibitors)
Amyloidosis	Acquired factor X deficiency, blood vessel infiltration

platelet disorders and congenital or acquired deficiency of coagulation factors, which can be confirmed by specific assay. The tests will not, however, detect all bleeding disorders, especially those due to vascular causes and mild von Willebrand's disease, and patients with a strong personal or family history of the condition, despite normal screening investigation, should be referred for special management.

Congenital disorders

Haemophilia A and B are rare conditions with a combined incidence of about 1:10 000 of the population. They are due to a deficiency of coagulation factors VIII (haemophilia A) and IX (haemophilia B). As the genes for both proteins are on the X chromosome, both haemophilias have sex linked inheritance—the daughters of a man with haemophilia are therefore obligate carriers. Patients with severe haemophilia (less than 2% factor VIII or IX) have spontaneous bleeding into muscles and joints that can lead to a crippling arthropathy. Patients with moderate (2-5%) and mild (>5%) conditions usually bleed only after trauma or surgery. Management is highly specialised and consists of preventing or treating bleeding episodes with plasma derived or recombinant clotting factors.

Von Willebrand's disease is a common bleeding disorder with an incidence of up to 1% in some populations. Most cases are mild, with bleeding only after a haemostatic challenge. Inheritance is autosomal dominant, with males and females equally affected. The condition is due to a reduction or structural abnormality of von Willebrand's factor, which has the dual role of promoting normal platelet function and stabilising coagulation factor VIII. Von Willebrand's disease can give normal results on screening tests, and diagnosis may require specialist investigation. Most patients with mild disease respond to desmopressin (DDAVP), but clotting factor concentrates are needed for a minority.

Acquired disorders

Most proteins of the coagulation cascade and their regulators and inhibitors necessary for haemostasis are synthesised in the liver. Acquired abnormalities can be due to impaired synthesis, increased consumption, or rarely the formation of autoantibodies against coagulation proteins. Liver disease can cause a severe bleeding disorder, with prolongation of the prothrombin time particularly, often with coexistent thrombocytopenia due to excessive pooling of platelets in an enlarged spleen. Malabsorption of vitamin K from the gut can cause a coagulation disorder similar to that caused by ingestion of warfarin. Disseminated intravascular coagulation is a rare cause of an acquired severe systemic failure of haemostasis with simultaneous microvascular thrombosis and generalised bleeding. Overwhelming bacterial infections—for example, meningococcal septicaemia or disseminated malignancies (such as prostatic, pancreatic, and acute promyelocytic leukaemia)—are the most common causes. Renal disease causes a variable bleeding disorder primarily due to platelet dysfunction; advancing age, prolonged use of steroids, and vitamin C deficiency can all result in excessive bruising. Abnormal bleeding has been reported with myeloproliferative, myelodysplastic, and lymphoproliferative disorders.

Thrombosis

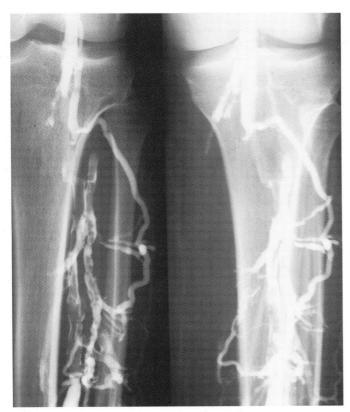

Figure 10.3 Contrast venogram showing extensive thrombosis with intraluminal filling defects and vessel occlusion.

Risk factors for venous thrombosis

Environmental
- Immobility
- Surgery, trauma
- Pregnancy, puerperium
- Long distance travel
- Use of combined oral contraceptives

Inherited
- Antithrombin deficiency
- Protein C deficiency
- Protein S deficiency
- Activated protein C resistance, factor V Leiden mutation

Acquired
- Antiphospholipid antibody, lupus anticoagulant
- Malignancy
- Myeloproliferative diseases

Clinical features of familial thrombophilia

- Family history of venous thromboembolism
- First episode at early age
- Recurrent venous thromboembolism
- Unusual site of thrombosis—for example, cerebral, mesenteric
- Thrombosis during pregnancy or puerperium
- Spontaneous venous thrombosis without environmental or acquired risk factor
- Recurrent superficial thrombophlebitis

Arterial thrombosis

Arterial thrombosis results in myocardial infarction, stroke, and peripheral vascular disease. Atherosclerotic lesions form in the vessel wall, resulting in narrowing and subsequent plaque rupture, which cause vessel occlusion. Risk factors for atherosclerosis include smoking, hypertension, diabetes, hypercholesterolaemia, hyperlipidaemia, and hyperfibrinogenaemia. Platelet deposition occurs on a ruptured arteriosclerotic plaque, and the antiplatelet drug aspirin is widely used in the treatment and secondary prophylaxis of arterial thrombosis.

Venous thrombosis

Venous thrombosis results in deep vein thrombosis and pulmonary embolism and is due to a combination of blood stasis and hypercoagulability. The clinical diagnosis of venous thromboembolic disease is notoriously unreliable, and objective confirmation with ultrasonography or venography for deep vein thrombosis and ventilation perfusion scanning or pulmonary angiography for pulmonary embolus must be performed. Recently it has become clear that venous thrombosis is frequently due to a combination of environmental factors (such as surgery and pregnancy), with an underlying genetic predisposition due to inherited deficiencies or abnormalities of the proteins of the natural anticoagulant pathway, which functions to inhibit or limit thrombin formation.

The incidence of the recently described condition activated protein C resistance is 3-5% in white populations, and it is thus the commonest cause of an inherited predisposition to venous thrombosis (thrombophilia), despite being rare in other ethnic groups. All the hereditary thrombophilic conditions are autosomally dominantly inherited and are present in up to 50% of cases of venous thrombosis, particularly when recurrent, familial, or at a young age. Detection of one of these conditions should not only influence the future management of the individual with regard to thromboprophylaxis and anticoagulation but also initiate family screening. Unfortunately the presence of active thrombosis and treatment with both heparin and warfarin make testing for the above conditions unreliable, and testing should be delayed until active thrombosis has resolved and anticoagulants have been discontinued, although the genetic test for the factor V Leiden defect is not affected.

An acquired predisposition to both arterial and venous thrombosis occurs in the antiphospholipid syndrome, which can either be primary or secondary to an underlying collagen vascular disorder. Laboratory diagnosis of this condition entails the detection of antibodies to cardiolipin or a lupus anticoagulant, or both. The latter causes in vitro a prolonged activated partial thromboplastin time and a prolonged dilute Russell's viper venom test, which corrects with excess phospholipids, but is paradoxically associated in vivo with thrombosis. Lupus anticoagulants can also be induced by infections and drugs, and in these circumstances are not usually associated with thrombosis.

Anticoagulation

Recommended international normalised ratio ranges

2·0-3·0

- Treatment of deep vein thrombosis and pulmonary embolism
- Atrial fibrillation
- Mitral stenosis with embolism
- Transient ischaemic attack

3·0-4·5

- Recurrence of deep vein thrombosis or pulmonary embolism while taking warfarin
- Mechanical prosthetic heart valves

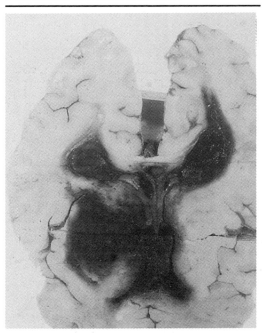

Figure 10.4 Intracerebral bleeding in patient taking warfarin

Reversal of oral anticoagulation

Condition	Treatment
INR >4·5 without bleeding	Stop warfarin transiently and review
INR >4·5 with minor bleeding	Stop warfarin and consider small doses of intravenous vitamin K
Life threatening bleeding	Stop warfarin; give intravenous vitamin K 5 mg; give factor II, IX, X, and VII concentrate (50 units/kg factor IX) if available (if concentrate is unavailable give 15-25 ml/kg fresh frozen plasma)
Unexpected bleeding at any INR	Consider unsuspected underlying structural lesion

INR = international normalised ratio

Warfarin

Warfarin is an oral anticoagulant that results in the synthesis by the liver of non-functional coagulation factors II, VII, IX, and X, as well as proteins C and S, by interfering with vitamin K metabolism.

Warfarin prolongs the prothrombin time, and dosage monitoring is achieved by a standardised form of this test, the international normalised ratio.

Recommended target ranges and duration of treatment have been published; an international normalised ratio of 2 to 3 is adequate for most cases.

Warfarin treatment requires regular monitoring as over-treatment carries an important haemorrhagic risk, and warfarin requirements may be affected by intercurrent illness or concurrent drug treatment. Dental extraction or minor surgery is usually safe if the international normalised ratio is less than 2·5, whereas for major surgery warfarin should be discontinued and parenteral heparin substituted.

In pregnancy warfarin is absolutely contraindicated from six to 12 weeks of gestation as it may damage the fetus. Because warfarin crosses the placenta and affects the fetus, heparin is increasingly being substituted throughout pregnancy as the drug of choice for thromboprophylaxis.

Reversal of a high international normalised ratio can be addressed in several ways, depending on the circumstances. In the absence of bleeding, omitting warfarin is usually sufficient. Minor bleeding episodes can be treated with local measures and small doses of vitamin K. Life threatening bleeding requires resuscitation of the patient together with treatment with coagulation factor concentrate; fresh frozen plasma can be used if concentrate is not available but is less effective.

Heparin

Heparin is a parenterally active anticoagulant that acts by potentiating the antithrombotic effects of antithrombin and can be used for both prophylaxis and treatment of venous thromboembolic disease. Unfractionated heparin is usually given intravenously and is monitored by prolongation of the activated partial thromboplastin time. It has a narrow therapeutic range with complex pharmacokinetics and great interpatient variation in dose requirements. Newer, low molecular weight heparins are replacing unfractionated heparin for both prophylaxis and treatment of venous thromboembolic disease. They can be administered by once daily subcutaneous injection without monitoring.

11 MALIGNANT LYMPHOMAS AND CHRONIC LYMPHOCYTIC LEUKAEMIA

G M Mead

> Management of the malignant lymphomas is complex and is best carried out in specialised treatment centres

The malignant lymphomas (non-Hodgkin's lymphoma and Hodgkin's disease) are a clinically and pathologically diverse group of cancers of largely unknown cause that are rapidly increasing in incidence. They are highly treatable and sometimes curable. Chronic lymphocytic leukaemia, the commonest adult leukaemia, shares many features with these cancers. The whole group constitutes about 5% of malignant diseases.

Pathology and staging

Ann Arbor staging system for lymphoma

Site
- Stage I—Single lymphoid area or extranodal site (stage IE)
- Stage II—Two lymphoid areas or extranodal sites on the same side of the diaphragm
- Stage III—Lymphoid areas (including the spleen) on both sides of the diaphragm
- Stage IV—Diffuse involvement of an extranodal organ(s) (liver, bone marrow)

Symptoms
- A—No symptoms
- B— >10% Weight loss, drenching night sweats, or unexplained fevers $\geqslant 38°C$

Binet staging system for chronic lymphocytic leukaemia

Stage A	No anaemia or thrombocytopenia; fewer than three enlarged lymphoid areas
Stage B	As for stage A but three or more enlarged lymphoid areas
Stage C	Anaemia (concentration <100 g/l) and/or platelet count $<100 \times 10^9$/l

The non-Hodgkin's lymphomas arise from malignant transformation of lymphocytes, deriving from B cells in about 85% of cases and T cells in most of the rest. Chronic lymphocytic leukaemia is largely a B cell malignancy, but the cell of origin of the Reed Sternberg cell, which characterises Hodgkin's disease, remains uncertain.

Histopathologically, lymphomas comprise an admixture of identical (monoclonal) malignant cells with variable amounts of reactive lymphoid cells and stroma. The lymphomas are variably subcategorised by pathologists into about 20 different types on the basis of conventional cytological staining and special stains to determine subtype and lineage.

A diagnosis of lymphoma (or even B or T cell lymphoma) gives no clue to the natural course of the disease in an individual patient. Clinicians treating these patients take account of the histopathology and the history provided by the patient, as well as many other factors (for example, stage and age), before recommending treatment or advising about prognosis. The complexity of non-Hodgkin's lymphomas requires a simplified management approach, on the basis of division of cases into low grade (or indolent), intermediate, and high grade disease.

All patients with lymphoma or chronic lymphocytic leukaemia require careful initial staging, usually comprising physical examination, computed tomography, and a bone marrow biopsy. Lymphomas are staged with the Ann Arbor system and chronic lymphocytic leukaemia with the Binet system. Increasingly, treatment is decided on the basis of allocated stage together with an examination of other known prognostic factors.

Low grade non-Hodgkin's lymphomas and chronic lymphocytic leukaemia

Presenting features of low grade non-Hodgkin's lymphoma

- Painless peripheral lymphadenopathy
- Abdominal mass (nodal or spleen)
- Weight loss
- Night sweats

Presenting features of chronic lymphocytic leukaemia

- As for low grade non-Hodgkin's lymphoma
- Asymptomatic—diagnosed coincidentally
- Fatigue
- Anaemia
- Infection

The low grade non-Hodgkin's lymphomas and chronic lymphocytic leukaemia are rare in patients aged under 40 years and are predominantly diseases of elderly people (90% of patients are aged >50 years).

Nodal non-Hodgkin's lymphomas and chronic lymphocytic leukaemia

This group includes most of the follicular lymphomas and constitutes about 30% of the cases of non-Hodgkin's lymphoma. Chronic lymphocytic leukaemia has a similar natural course. Diagnosis may be incidental (for example, from a routine blood count, as in chronic lymphocytic leukaemia) or may follow a period of (often fluctuating) localised or generalised enlargement of lymph nodes or the spleen. These lymphomas are usually widespread at diagnosis, commonly (as in non-Hodgkin's lymphoma) or always (chronic lymphocytic leukaemia)

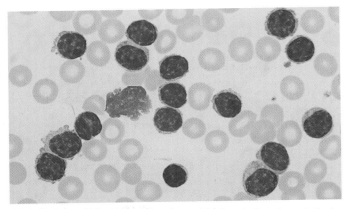

Figure 11.1 Peripheral blood film of patient with chronic lymphocytic leukaemia showing numerous malignant lymphocytes.

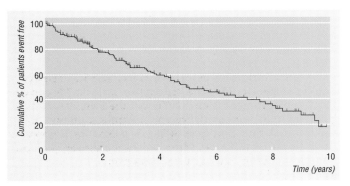

Figure 11.2 Survival curve of 160 patients with advanced follicular lymphoma: survival is prolonged, but there is no evidence of cure.

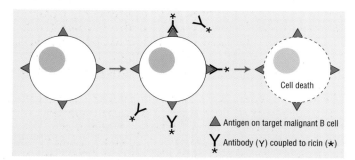

Figure 11.3 "Targeted" antibody therapy of lymphoma. The antibody delivers a toxin (ricin) to the lymphocytes bearing the appropriate surface antigen.

involving the bone marrow. Because of their indolent nature, however, there may be little or no initial effect on quality of life. Some patients, however, present with B symptoms or bulky widespread disease and need early treatment.

The management of these cancers is adjusted to their natural course. Cure can rarely be achieved, and the median overall survival in most series is five to eight years. Prognosis relates to age (poorer when older) and particularly to the extent of disease judged in terms of bulk and effect of tumour. The outlook for chronic lymphocytic leukaemia worsens with increasing extent of disease at presentation and cytopenias (Binet stage B and C).

Patients who are well with non-threatening disease may initially be watched without treatment—on occasions for many years. Initial treatment when needed generally comprises an alkylating agent—usually intermittent chlorambucil—with or without steroids for four to six months and will often be highly successful in causing disease regression; relapse is, however, inevitable. After several years these lymphomas may become refractory to treatment or may "transform" with change in histology and clinical course to an intermediate grade non-Hodgkin's lymphoma. If this occurs then combination chemotherapy is recommended, but the outlook is usually poor.

Promising new treatments that are being evaluated include fludarabine, a new chemotherapy agent, and antibody treatment. Monoclonal antibodies directed against B cell antigens may be used alone or coupled to a toxin (or therapeutic dose of a radio isotope) and can "target" the malignant lymphoid cell. High dose therapy with stem cell rescue is also used.

Extranodal lymphoma (maltoma)

The maltomas (mucosal associated lymphoid tumours) were first described about 15 years ago. These are indolent lymphomas that arise most commonly in the stomach, thyroid, parotid, and lung—often evolving from a pre-existing inflammatory or autoimmune disease (for example, gastritis related to *Helicobacter pylori* or Sjögren's syndrome). These tumours have been successfully managed with local resection or radiotherapy, or both. There is, however, increasing evidence suggesting that gastric maltoma can be controlled or cured by use of appropriate antibiotics, a highly unusual example of malignant regression by treatment of infection.

The maltomas can progress to intermediate grade tumours. In addition they can metastasise, usually to the other maltoma sites described above.

Intermediate grade non-Hodgkin's lymphoma

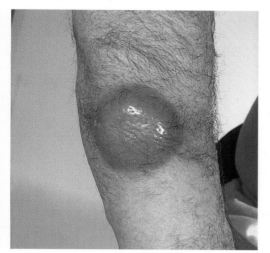

Figure 11.4 Intermediate grade non-Hodgkin's lymphoma arising in skin.

This is the most common grade of non-Hodgkin's lymphoma (65%) and affects any age group. It is rapidly increasing in incidence, although the reasons for this are uncertain. Two thirds of cases of this type of cancer arise within lymph nodes—patients present because of lymph node enlargement. The remaining cases may arise in almost any other tissue or organ (for example, gastrointestinal tract, skin, brain, and bone), with symptoms appropriate to each site.

The most common type is diffuse large cell lymphoma, a B cell neoplasm. These lymphomas occur at any age (median 65 years) and are rapidly progressive cancers that are often associated with B symptoms. Diagnosis and staging should be urgently performed then treatment with chemotherapy started. These are curable cancers in about 40% of cases. The prognosis relates to the patient's age, extent of spread, lactate dehydrogenase concentration, and performance status.

The standard chemotherapy is a combination of cyclophosphamide, doxorubicin, vincristine, and prednisolone (CHOP) given intravenously at intervals of three weeks in outpatient clinics on six occasions and sometimes supplemented by radiotherapy.

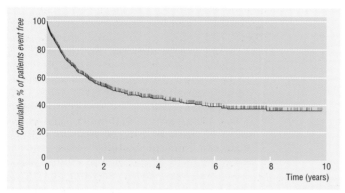

Figure 11.5 Survival of 760 patients with large cell non-Hodgkin's lymphoma (40% cure rate).

Relapse is not uncommon and in the past was associated with a poor outlook. However, younger patients with disease that has remained sensitive to chemotherapy may now be cured in up to 50% of cases using high dose chemotherapy. Survival in remaining patients is often measurable in months.

High grade non-Hodgkin's lymphoma

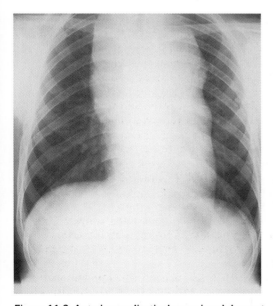

Figure 11.6 Anterior mediastinal mass in adolescent male: histological tests revealed lymphoblastic lymphoma.

This grade of the disease is rare (under 5% of all cases) and comprises rapidly progressive cancers of children and young adults.

Lymphoblastic lymphoma is a T cell lymphoma predominantly of young males that usually presents with a mediastinal mass. Involvement of the bone marrow and central nervous system commonly occur. Burkitt's lymphoma as seen in Europe and America is a rare B cell neoplasm of young adults that usually arises at extranodal sites most commonly in the gastrointestinal tract-for example, the ileocaecal region. This lymphoma also commonly spreads to the bone marrow and the central nervous system.

Both these lymphoma types are curable with intensive combination chemotherapy; the role of high dose therapy is under evaluation.

Treatment of these cancers is urgent and may, if adequate precautions are not taken, be complicated by the acute tumour lysis syndrome resulting from breakdown of the lymphoma. This can lead to renal failure and possible death. Prophylaxis against relapse in the central nervous system is routinely used. Overall cure rates generally exceed 50%.

AIDS related non-Hodgkin's lymphoma

Treatment of AIDS related non-Hodgkin's lymphoma

- Treatment is often difficult because of pre-existing immunosuppression and AIDS related infection
- Chemotherapy is usually indicated; the prognosis relates to the degree of immunosuppression at diagnosis
- Cure of these lymphomas is possible, although the outlook is usually very poor

The immunosuppression associated with HIV infection has been associated with a noticeable increase in the incidence of non-Hodgkin's lymphoma and Hodgkin's disease.

These diseases arise in many cases because of uninhibited expansion of multiple clones of lymphocytes infected with Epstein-Barr virus. They are commonly high grade B cell neoplasms that arise at extranodal sites—for example, the brain and the ileocaecal area.

Hodgkin's disease

> Hodgkin's disease is an uncommon form of lymphoma occurring mainly at ages 15-35 years and affects slightly more men than women

Symptoms and signs of Hodgkin's disease

- Painless lymphadenopathy
- B symptoms
- Pruritus

Clinical features of Hodgkin's disease v non-Hodgkin's lymphoma

	Hodgkin's disease	Non-Hodgkin's lymphoma
Incidence	Stable	Increasing
Age	Median 29 years	Increasing incidence with age
Sites	Nodal; supradiaphragmatic	Nodal or extranodal; any site
Clinical features	Mediastinal mass; itching; alcohol induced pain	Nil specific
Prognosis	70-80% cure	Highly variable by type; most incurable

Pathology

Hodgkin's disease has classically been divided into four types. Recent studies suggest, however, that one type—lymphocyte predominance—is a clinically distinct B cell lymphoma often presenting with isolated enlargement of a peripheral lymph node.

The nodular sclerosing type constitutes 70-80% of cases of Hodgkin's disease and classically presents in young women with mediastinal and cervical nodal disease.

Mixed cellularity disease occurs predominantly in older males and is more commonly widespread. Lymphocyte depleted Hodgkin's disease is rare.

Clinical presentation and management

Hodgkin's disease most commonly presents as enlargement of supradiaphragmatic lymph nodes with or without B symptoms. Generalised pruritus can be a presenting feature in some cases. The spleen is involved in at least 30% of cases, and in the past the disease was detected with splenectomy. This procedure has now been abandoned as studies suggested no overall survival benefit from this procedure, and modern management instead relies on assessment of prognostic factors—which are used to assess the likelihood of early stage disease being encompassed by radiotherapy with a reasonable chance of cure. Staging is, as for non-Hodgkin's lymphoma, with the Ann Arbor system.

Patients with early stage disease (non-bulky stage I and IIA) are managed with radiotherapy. Treatment confined to the involved area is used for localised lymphocyte predominant disease. The remaining cases receive at least mantle radiotherapy (treatment of bilateral cervical and axillary nodes combined with treatment to the mediastinum), resulting in cure in 60-70% of cases. Patients with more extensive or symptomatic disease and those for whom initial radiotherapy fails receive combination chemotherapy incorporating doxorubicin. About two thirds of patients receiving chemotherapy will remain permanently free of disease as a result of this treatment. At the time of relapse treatment may comprise further chemotherapy or high dose chemotherapy with peripheral stem cell rescue-radiotherapy often also has a role.

Long term studies suggest that the overall cure rates for Hodgkin's disease are stable at 70-80%, although it is hoped that high dose chemotherapy may improve these figures. In the past chemotherapy was invariably associated with infertility and premature menopause-newer treatments carry much less risk of these problems. Late toxicity—particularly second malignancy—remains the source of concern in patients that have been treated with wide field radiotherapy or chemotherapy. Patients with early stage disease are increasingly being managed with limited radiation fields combined with brief courses of chemotherapy in an attempt to avoid this complication.

Dr Dina Choudhury provided the blood film showing chronic lymphocytic leukaemia.

Further reading

- O'Brien S, del Giglio A, Keating M. Advances in the biology and treatment of B-cell chronic lymphocytic leukemia. *Blood* 1995;85:307-18.
- Aisenberg AC. Coherent view of non-Hodgkin's lymphoma. *J Clin Oncol* 1995;13:2656-75.
- DeVita VT, Hubbard SM. Hodgkin's disease. *N Engl J Med* 1993;328:560-5.

12 BONE MARROW AND STEM CELL TRANSPLANTATION

Andrew Duncombe

History

> Early animal studies of bone marrow transplantation were translated into clinical practice with understanding of the human leucocyte antigen (HLA) system and immunosuppressive therapy

Experiments in the 1950s showed that haemopoiesis could be restored in irradiated animals by engraftment of transfused marrow. Attempts to translate this into clinical practice were hindered by immunological problems of transfer between individuals which we now recognise as rejection and graft versus host disease.

With further understanding of the human leucocyte antigen system, rapid clinical progress was made during the 1970s such that bone marrow transplantation soon became an established treatment for some immune deficiency and malignant diseases.

What is a bone marrow transplant?

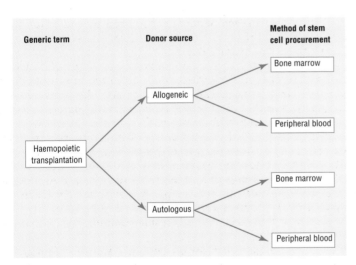

Figure 12.1 Transplant terminology.

> The aim of haemopoietic transplantation is the elimination of the underlying disease in the recipient, together with full restoration of haemopoietic and immune function

Transplantation is the reconstitution of the full haemopoietic system by transfer of the pluripotent cells present in the bone marrow (stem cells). This usually requires prior ablation of the patient's own marrow by intensive chemotherapy or chemoradiotherapy.

The most appropriate generic term for the procedure is haemopoietic transplantation, which may be subdivided according to the donor source and further subdivided into the site of stem cell procurement.

Allogeneic transplantation is when another individual acts as the donor-usually a sibling of the patient, sometimes a normal volunteer. All cases, however, require a full or near HLA match—that is, they should be HLA compatible. Autologous transplantation is when the patient acts as his or her own source of stem cells.

Originally, stem cells were procured from the bone marrow by direct puncture and aspiration of bone marrow and reinfused intravenously, a procedure known as bone marrow transplantation. Recently, it has been shown that stem cells derived from the bone marrow can be liberated into the peripheral blood, where the cells are harvested with a cell separation machine. Transplant operations with this stem cell material are known as peripheral blood stem cell transplantations. Stem cells derived from the bone marrow or peripheral blood may be used in either an allogeneic or an autologous setting.

Allogeneic transplantation

Indications for allogeneic transplantation

When it is sole chance of cure
- Primary immunodeficiency syndromes
- Aplastic anaemia
- Thalassaemia
- Sickle cell disease
- Inborn errors of metabolism
- Chronic myeloid leukaemia

When it substantially increases chances of cure
- Acute myeloid leukaemia (first or second complete remission)
- Acute lymphoblastic leukaemia (first or second full remission)*
- Myelodysplasia
- Multiple myeloma

* In children, in whom acute lymphoblastic leukaemia is the commonest leukaemia, most will be cured by standard chemotherapy alone, without transplantation (which is reserved for those who relapse)

> Although the size of bone marrow registries is increasing, the heterogeneity of the HLA complex means that there is still a shortage of appropriately matched donors for all potential recipients

Suitability

Owing to the profound toxicity of the transplant procedure potential recipients should be otherwise healthy and aged <55 years. As bone marrow contains B and T lymphocytes along with macrophages the donor and recipient must be fully or near fully HLA matched to prevent life threatening graft versus host disease or rejection.

This restricts the availability of potential donors. Within the patient's family the greatest chance of a full HLA match is with a sibling. An average recipient in Western countries has about a 1 in 4 chance of having a sibling who is fully HLA matched.

With this restriction in allogeneic transplantation, interest has surrounded the use of normal volunteer donors who show a close HLA match to the potential recipient. This has been achieved by the establishment of bone marrow registries in which volunteers agree to donate marrow. There are two such registries in Britain—the National Blood Transfusion Service and the Anthony Nolan panels.

Autologous transplantation

Indications for autologous transplantation

Proved benefit in randomised controlled trials
- Relapsed non-Hodgkin's lymphoma (intermediate and high grade)
- Acute myeloid leukaemia (first or second complete remission)
- Multiple myeloma

Probable benefit
- Relapsed Hodgkin's disease
- Acute lymphoblastic leukaemia in adults (first or second complete remission)
- Relapsed testicular cancer

Possible benefit
- Chronic myeloid leukaemia
- Disseminated breast cancer
- Disseminated lung cancers
- Other solid tumours
- Severe autoimmune disease

Suitability

Less immunological disturbance occurs in autologous than in allogeneic transplantation as the donor and the recipient are the same individual; the stresses on the cardiorespiratory, skin, and mucosal systems, however, are similar. Autologous recipients therefore should still be otherwise healthy but can be aged up to about 70 years.

Indications

These are being continuously evaluated by a number of studies including randomised control trials in many diseases, particularly malignancy. The indications can best be broken down into those in which there is now proved benefit in randomised controlled trials, those in which there is probable benefit, and those in which there is possible benefit.

Obtaining the graft

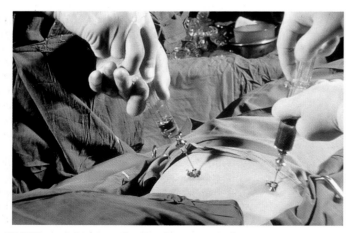

Figure 12.2 Haematologists performing bone marrow harvest.

Bone marrow is harvested by puncture of the iliac crests under general anaesthesia. It is aspirated directly from the marrow cavity with marrow biopsy needles.

Up to a litre of marrow may be needed to provide sufficient stem cells for transplantation. The procedure is well tolerated, requiring only simple analgesia postoperatively. Serious complications are rare.

In peripheral blood stem cell transplantations, stem cells are mobilised into the blood by single agent chemotherapy or a haemopoietic growth factor (for example, granulocyte colony stimulating factor), or both. When the white blood count rises after 5-12 days, the individual is connected to a cell separation machine, blood is drawn off and spun in a centrifuge, and stem cells are harvested while the remaining blood elements are returned to the patient. The procedure takes 2-4 hours and is well tolerated.

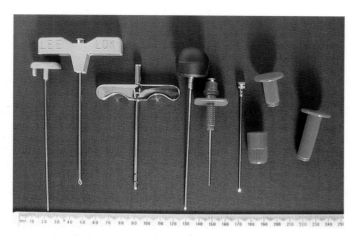

Figure 12.3 Needles for bone marrow harvesting.

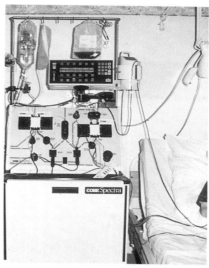

Figure 12.4 Extracorporeal cell separation device for collection of peripheral blood stem cells, showing inlet and outlet intravenous lines; collected stem cell product is in bag above machine.

Peripheral blood stem cell transplantation is gradually replacing bone marrow transplantation as the procedure of choice as no general anaesthesia is needed, engraftment is more rapid with earlier discharge from hospital, and the procedure is cheaper.

Transplantation procedures

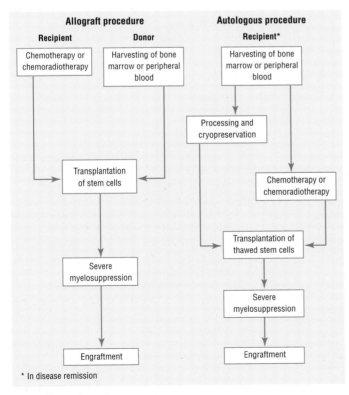

Figure 12.5 Transplantation procedures.

Allogeneic transplantation

The recipient is treated with high dose chemotherapy or chemoradiotherapy to ablate the bone marrow (conditioning). On the day after the treatment has ended, bone marrow or peripheral blood stem cells are harvested from the donor, and the transplant is performed by infusing the stem cells intravenously. After a period of severe myelosuppression lasting 7-21 days, engraftment of the transplanted material takes place. Full engraftment may not be complete for several months.

Autologous transplantation

The recipient, while in disease remission, undergoes a bone marrow or peripheral blood stem cell harvest. The stem cells are processed and frozen in liquid nitrogen. The recipient then starts conditioning. One day after the conditioning has ended, the stem cell product is thawed and infused intravenously. The bags are thawed rapidly by transfer directly from a liquid nitrogen container into water at 37-43°C. The product is infused intravenously rapidly through an indwelling central line. Myelosuppression and engraftment follow as described above.

One major procedural difference between allogeneic and autologous transplantation is the requirement for immunosuppression in allografts to prevent graft versus host disease and rejection. This is achieved with combinations of cyclosporin A and methotrexate or with in vitro or in vivo depletion of T cells using monoclonal antibodies.

Procedural complications

Early complications of transplants

Chemoradiotherapy
- Nausea and vomiting
- Reversible alopecia
- Fatigue
- Dry inflamed skin
- Mucositis
- Veno-occlusive disease

Infections
- Bacterial (Gram negative and positive)
- Viral—herpes zoster virus, cytomegalovirus (particularly pneumonitis)
- Fungi—candida, aspergillus
- Atypical organisms—pneumocystis pneumonia, toxoplasma, mycoplasma, legionella

Acute graft versus host disease (allograft only)
- Rash
- Diarrhoea
- Jaundice

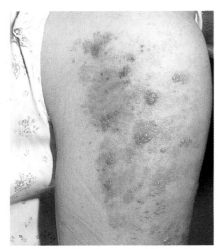

Figure 12.6 Severe herpes zoster on upper arm after transplant.

Clinical features of graft versus host disease

Acute
- Skin rash (typically palms and soles)
- Abdominal pain
- Profuse diarrhoea
- Jaundice (intrahepatic cholestasis)

Chronic
- Sclerotic atrophic skin
- Sicca syndrome
- Mucosal ulceration
- Malabsorption syndromes
- Recurrent chest infections
- Cholestatic jaundice
- Joint movement restriction
- Hyposplenic infections—for example, pneumococcus
- Myelosuppression

Late complications of transplantation

- Relapse of the original underlying disease
- Infertility (both sexes)
- Hypothyroidism
- Secondary malignancy
- Late sepsis due to hyposplenism
- Cataracts (secondary to total body irradiation)
- Psychological disturbance

Early complications

Allogeneic and autologous procedures are associated with considerable morbidity and mortality. Overall, transplant related mortality for autologous recipients is 2–15%, for recipients of sibling HLA matched allografts 15-30%, and for recipients of allografts from volunteer, unrelated donors up to 45%.

Nausea and vomiting from chemoradiotherapy is controllable with drugs, but the widespread mucosal damage to the gastrointestinal tract causes mucositis, which can be more difficult to control. Oral ulceration, buccal desquamation, oesophagitis, gastritis, abdominal pain, and diarrhoea may all be features.

The severe myelosuppression after the transplant, together with immune dysfunction from delayed reconstitution or graft versus host disease, predisposes to a wide variety of potentially fatal infections with bacterial (Gram positive and negative), viral, fungal, and atypical organisms. Prophylactic antibiotics may reduce their incidence, but astute surveillance and prompt intervention with intravenous antibiotics are mandatory.

Infection with the herpes simplex virus or the herpes zoster virus is common, and infection with the herpes zoster virus in particular may present with fulminant extensive lesions.

The most feared viral infection after allografting, however, is caused by cytomegalovirus. This may give rise to fulminant cytomegalovirus pneumonitis, which still has a high mortality despite newer antiviral drugs.

Fungal infections with candida species are common, and disseminated aspergillus infection is particularly serious. Preventive measures include the use of broad spectrum antifungal agents prophylactically and the use of air filtration in positive pressure isolation cubicles for patients throughout transplant.

Graft versus host disease is classified as acute if occurring within 100 days of transplantation and chronic if occurring after that time. Acute graft versus host disease ranges from a mild self limiting condition to a fatal disorder. The mainstay of treatment remains steroids, but severe disease resistant to steroids is usually fatal. Chronic graft versus host disease is associated with collagen deposition and sclerotic change in the skin, giving a wider distribution of affected organs than the acute disease. Treatment is with combinations of cyclosporin and prednisolone aimed at controlling disease and ameliorating symptoms.

Follow up treatment and surveillance

Cost of haemopoietic transplants

- Haemopoietic transplants score highly on quality of life adjusted years (QALY) analysis, and the cost per QALY is low
- The cost for each patient will depend on the disease, type of transplant, and particularly on whether complications occur
- A typical cost for one patient is £15 000-£65 000
- A successful allogeneic transplant for thalassaemia or primary immunodeficiency will prevent expensive, lifelong alternative supportive treatment
- The cost of transplantation in malignant disease must be offset against the substantial costs of ongoing alternative chemotherapy

For allograft recipients, immunosuppression needs careful monitoring to avoid toxicity. Unlike transplant recipients of solid organs, recipients of haemopoietic transplants do not need lifelong immunosuppression, and cyclosporin is normally discontinued about six months after transplantation. Prophylactic prescription for specific infections is required including penicillin to prevent pneumococcal sepsis secondary to hyposplenism, aciclovir to prevent reactivation of the herpes simplex virus and the herpes zoster virus, and co-trimoxazole or pentamidine to prevent infection with *Pneumocystis carinii*.

Regular haematological follow up is mandatory, and psychological support from the transplant team, family, and friends is vital for readjustment to normal life. Expert counselling and psychiatric input may occasionally be needed.

Despite all the above potential complications most patients return to an active, working life without continuing treatment.

The future

Future developments in haemopoietic transplantation

- Improved DNA matching techniques for volunteer, unrelated donors
- Rapid matching on the Internet
- Umbilical cord blood as transplant source
- Gene therapy (in haemophilia, haemoglobinopathy, and cystic fibrosis)

Haemopoietic transplantation is an exciting and rapidly developing field—with the techniques being applied to broader categories of disease, such as autoimmune diseases, as well as being the vehicle for future gene therapy (for example, haemophilia and thalassaemia). The haemopoietic stem cell's property of infinite self renewal makes it an ideal target vehicle for insertion of genes. Candidates include factor VIII gene replacement in haemophilia. The molecular revolution has already resulted in greatly improved DNA matching at the HLA gene loci, which should ensure greater applicability and success of transplants from volunteer unrelated donors. Registration and matching from banks of volunteer donors and umbilical cord donors will be accelerated by the use of the Internet, enabling wider and speedier access of potential grafts to recipients in need.

Some of the photographs were provided by Dr J Treleaven and Mr R Smith.

13   HAEMATOLOGICAL DISORDERS AT THE EXTREMES OF LIFE

Adrian C Newland, Tyrrell G J R Evans

Infants

Common causes of anaemia in newborn infants

- Blood loss—Occult bleeding (fetomaternal, fetoplacental, twin to twin); obstetric accidents; internal bleeding; iatrogenic
- Increased destruction—Immune haemolytic anaemia; infection; haemoglobinopathies; enzymopathies
- Decreased production—infection; nutritional deficiencies

Anaemia in neonates

The haemoglobin concentration at birth is 159-191 g/l. It rises transiently in the first 24 hours but then slowly falls to as low as 95 g/l by 9 weeks. By 6 months, the concentration stabilises at around 125 g/l, the lower end of the adult range, increasing towards adolescence. The normal fall in haemoglobin concentration seen in full term infants is accentuated in prematurity and may fall to less than 90 g/l by 4 weeks. Preterm infants are particularly prone to multiple nutritional deficiencies because of rapid growth. Pronounced anaemia may be assumed if the infant gains insufficient weight or is fatigued while feeding.

Normal haematology values in newborn infants

	Haemoglobin (g/l)	Red blood cells ($\times 10^{12}$/l)	Mean cell volume (fl)	Nucleated red blood cells (per ml)
Day 1	168-212	4·44-5·84	109·6-128·4	500
Week 1	150-196	4·0-5·6	93·0-131·0	0
Week 4	111-143	3·2-4·0	92·9-109·1	0
Week 8	98-116	2·9-3·9	105·0-81·0	0
Week 12	104-122	3·4-4·0	80·1-95·9	0

Haemolytic disease in newborn infants

Recommendations for prophylactic anti-D immunoglobulin in RhD negative women
- After delivery if the infant is Rh positive
- After abortion (therapeutic or spontaneous)
- To cover antenatal procedures (amniocentesis, chorionic villus sampling)
- After threatened abortion or miscarriage
- Antenatally at 28 and 34 weeks (not yet universal)

Reasons for failure of prophylaxis
- Failure of administration (commonest cause)
- Inadequate dosage (routine Kleihauer tests should be performed)
- Earlier sensitisation that may not be detectable at birth
- Poor injection technique (should be deep intramuscular)

Haemolytic disease in newborn infants

Haemolytic disease in newborn infants is due to destruction of fetal red cells by antibodies from the mother that cross the placenta. The most important are antibodies to the RhD antigen. Maternal immunisation is preventable by the prophylactic use of anti-D immunoglobulin, and since its introduction in the 1960s the number of affected babies has fallen dramatically. Anti-D immunoglobulin is administered to non-sensitised RhD negative women, but prophylaxis may fail.

In severely affected fetuses, mortality used to be as high as 40%, with only exchange transfusion available after delivery to correct anaemia and prevent kernicterus. Intrauterine transfusion, initially via the intraperitoneal route, was introduced to prevent problems in the fetus. However, it was the development in the early 1980s of intravascular blood transfusion using fetoscopy into the umbilical artery that dramatically improved survival. Hydrops can be readily reversed in utero, and even in the most severe group the survival rate has been 85%.

HIV infection

- HIV may produce a chronic multisystem disease in children
- Perinatal transmission of the virus from an infected woman is the primary route of exposure to the fetus (20-40% of pregnancies)
- Thrombocytopenia occurs in up to 15% of children with HIV infection
- Anaemia is also common, occurring early, usually with the normocytic, normochromic features of chronic disease
- Leucopenia and lymphopenia are also seen, in which the bone marrow shows non-specific features of chronic infection

Anaemia associated with infection

Cytomegalovirus, rubella, toxoplasmosis, and more rarely congenital syphilis may be associated with anaemia due either to haemolysis or to bone marrow suppression. More recently human parvovirus B19 has been identified as a cause of anaemia and fetal damage. In early pregnancy maternal infection may lead to spontaneous abortion, but in later pregnancy it may lead to selective depression of erythropoiesis with profound anaemia and

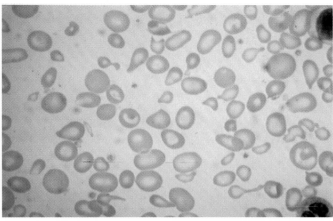

Figure 13.1 Peripheral blood of patient with Hb H disease showing pale red cells (hypochromia) with variation in size and shape (anisopoikilocystois).

Features of α thalassaemia

Syndrome	Haematological abnormalities	Diagnosis
Silent carrier (- α/α α)*	No anaemia or microcytosis	1-2% Hb Bart's†
Thalassaemia trait (- α/- α)	Mild anaemia and microcytosis	3-10% Hb Bart's
Hb H disease (- -/- α)	Moderate microcytic, hypochromic haemolytic anaemia	20-40% Hb Bart's
Hb Bart's hydrops syndrome (- -/- -)	Severe microcytic hypochromic anaemia (lethal)	80% Hb Bart's, 20% Hb H‡

* Where α α/α α is normal (that is, 4 α genes) and - α represents deletion of one α gene on a chromosome
† Bart's γ_4 tetramers
‡ Hb H β_4 tetramers

Antenatal screening for carrier detection of sickle cell disease (with subsequent study of the partners of positive women) should be carried out so that prenatal diagnosis can be offered

In up to 30% of all new cases patients will have no family history of coagulation disorders, and such cases are therefore new mutations

the development of hydrops. It may also induce an aplastic crisis or chronic haemolysis in normal children but is a major problem in those with an underlying haemoglobinopathy.

Malaria is a major health hazard worldwide, and easier travel to endemic areas has increased the problem. Inadequate or non-existent prophylaxis has led to an increase in cases over the past few years; unsuspected infection in neonates, usually caught from the mother, may be associated with a high mortality.

The haemoglobinopathies

β Thalassaemia major is an inherited haemoglobin disorder caused by reduction in β globin chain synthesis. It affects primarily people from the Indian subcontinent and of Mediterranean origin. It presents during the first year of life after the switch from fetal to adult haemoglobin. If production of the latter is reduced, anaemia occurs. The infant presents with failure to thrive, poor weight gain, feeding problems, and irritability. The blood appearances are typical, with severe anaemia associated with microcytosis and hypochromia with pronounced morphological change in the red cells. The infant will be dependent on transfusions unless bone marrow transplantation is feasible. The carrier state (thalassaemia minor or thalassaemia trait) mimics iron deficiency, from which it must be differentiated.

α Thalassaemia presents a similar picture and is a common cause of stillbirth in South East Asia.

Sickle cell disease

Sickle cell disease is caused by a structural abnormality of the β chain and is associated with a steady state haemoglobin of 50-110 g/l. In homozygous sickle cell disease the haemoglobin forms crystals, distorting the red blood cells into a rigid sickle cell shape. It is these sickle cells that block the microvasculature causing sickle cell crises. Mortality and morbidity are increased at all ages, with the peak incidence of death at age 1-3 years. Sickle cell crises are precipitated by infection, hypoxia, dehydration, cold, and exhaustion and are particularly common in adverse environmental or poor socioeconomic conditions. In infants, crises present with the clinical problems of infection, splenic sequestration, and dactylitis. Towards the end of the first year, painful vaso-occlusive crises are more common, and pneumococcal septicaemia related to splenic dysfunction is particularly apparent.

Genetic counselling and prenatal diagnosis have made an important contribution to reducing the number of affected children in countries with a comprehensive screening programme.

Disorders of haemostasis

Deficiencies of clotting factor VIII (haemophilia A) or factor IX (haemophilia B or Christmas disease) may present symptomatically in the first days of life with spontaneous bleeding. Bleeding from the cord or intracranial haemorrhage, however, are fortunately rare. Severe bleeding usually occurs at, for example, circumcision or when mobility increases. Both disorders of coagulation affect 1 in 10 000 of the population. They are X linked and clinically indistinguishable. The diagnosis may be suspected from the family history and can be confirmed antenatally.

Common causes of thrombocytopenia

- Immune mediated
    - Neonatal alloimmune thrombocytopenia
    - Maternal immune thrombocytopenia purpura
    - Drug induced
- Infection
    - Viral—for example, cytomegalovirus, HIV, rubella
    - Toxoplasmosis
- Post exchange transfusion
- Disorders of haemostasis
    - Disseminated intravascular coagulation
    - Maternal pre-eclampsia
    - Rhesus isoimmunisation
    - Hypothermia, hypoxia
    - Type IIB von Willebrand's disease
- Liver disease
- Giant haemangioma
- Hereditary thrombocytopenia
- Marrow infiltration

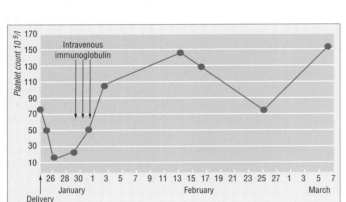

Figure 13.2 Response of neonate to intravenous immunoglobulin with thrombocytopenia secondary to maternal immune thrombocytopenia purpura.

Haemorrhagic disease of newborn infants

Type	Clinical signs	Causes
Early (within 24 hours)	Severe bleeding, often internal	Mother receiving drugs affecting vitamin K—eg, anticonvulsant (phenytoin), warfarin, antituberculosis drugs (rifampicin, isoniazid)
Classic (2-5 days)	Bruising or bleeding from gastrointestinal tract or after circumcision	Breast feeding, full term
Delayed (up to 1 month)	Intracranial haemorrhage, common	Prolonged breast feeding without prophylaxis; chronic diarrhoea, malabsorption, or oral antibiotics

Thrombocytopenia

Healthy infants have a platelet count in the adult range $(150\text{-}400 \times 10^9/l)$. Thrombocytopenia is the most common haemostatic abnormality in newborn infants, occurring in up to a quarter of babies admitted to neonatal intensive treatment units. Asphyxia at birth, infection, and disseminated intravascular coagulation are the most common causes of thrombocytopenia. It may also occur after exchange transfusion. Platelet transfusions should be given to any infant whose count is $< 20 \times 10^9/l$.

Maternal autoimmune thrombocytopenia may be associated with neonatal thrombocytopenia because of placental transfer of antiplatelet antibodies. Fetal platelet counts rarely drop below $50 \times 10^9/l$, and intracranial haemorrhage is rare either prenatally or at birth. However, the count may fall in the first few days of life, and treatment may be needed at this stage.

There are no reliable predictors of severe thrombocytopenia. Treatment includes platelet transfusions and corticosteroids, but intravenous immunoglobulin is safe and effective in over 80% of infants.

Neonatal alloimmune thrombocytopenia is associated with severe thrombocytopenia, and intracranial haemorrhage is seen in up to 15% of infants. Maternal platelet counts are normal, and maternal alloantibodies are directed against paternally derived antigens on the infant's platelets (usually HPA-1). In at risk pregnancies fetal blood sampling by cordocentesis should be used to confirm the HPA-1 status. Treatment relies on platelet transfusions in utero, but high dose intravenous immunoglobulin may be of some benefit.

Vitamin K deficiency

Haemorrhagic disease in newborn infants may be associated with vitamin K deficiency. It may be seen in otherwise healthy term infants especially if they are being breast fed. The deficiency may be precipitated if the mother is taking anticonvulsant drugs or warfarin. It may present soon after birth with generalised bruising and internal bleeding or as late as age 1 month.

Treatment is now aimed at prevention by administering vitamin K prophylaxis, although some controversy remains about whether this should be given orally or parenterally.

Elderly people

The possibility of an occult gastrointestinal malignancy (for example, caecal carcinoma) leading to iron deficiency anaemia should be considered

Haemoglobin concentration gradually declines from age 60 years, with a more rapid fall over the age of 70. The fall is accompanied, however, by a widening of the reference range, such that age dependent ranges are of little value in individuals.

Concentration should be considered in association with the clinical history. In older patients the lower end of the normal range should be reduced to 110 g/l.

Iron deficiency anaemias

Between 10% and 20% of old people will be anaemic, usually with iron deficiency. In many this will be nutritional, owing to difficulties in obtaining and eating food, for both medical and social reasons. Aspirin

Clinical associations in iron deficiency

Symptoms—Lethargy, lassitude, reduced activity; shortness of breath; angina on effort; intermittent claudication
Signs—Pallor, peripheral oedema; brittle nails, koilonychia; glossitis; stomatitis
Other gastrointestinal findings—Oesophageal web; atrophic gastritis; subtotal villous atrophy with malabsorption

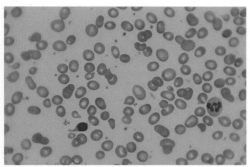

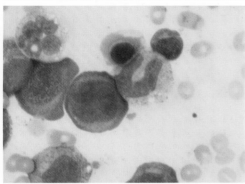

Figure 13.3 Megaloblastic anaemia: peripheral blood (top) showing macrocytes, tear drops, and multisegmented neutrophils; megaloblastic bone marrow (bottom) showing megaloblasts, giant metamyelocytes, and hypersegmented neutrophil.

Findings in anaemia of chronic disease

- Mild normocytic or microcytic anaemia
- Low serum iron concentration and iron binding capacity
- Reduced transferrin saturation
- Normal or raised serum ferritin concentration
- Increased iron in reticuloendothelial stores—for example, bone marrow
- Defective iron transfer to red cell precursors
- Iron reduced in red cell precursors
- Increased red cell protoporphyrin

Screening tests in anaemia of chronic disease*

- Review of peripheral blood film
- Erythrocyte sedimentation rate
- Liver and renal screen
- Chest radiograph
- Autoantibody screen
- Urine analysis
- Thyroid function studies
- Tumour markers
  Immunoglobulins (myeloma)
  Prostate specific antigen
  α Fetoprotein (liver)
  Carcinoembryonic antigen (gastrointestinal)

* After history and clinical examination

or non-steroidal anti-inflammatory drugs leading to occult gastrointestinal blood loss may also contribute. The problem may also be exacerbated in elderly people as gastric atrophy may occur, leading to poor absorption of iron supplements.

Oral supplements are usually well tolerated and should be continued for three months after the haemoglobin concentration has returned to normal, to replenish the iron stores.

Megaloblastic anaemia

Folic acid deficiency also occurs readily in those who eat poorly and can be easily corrected by supplements. Pernicious anaemia due to vitamin B12 deficiency also occurs in middle and later life and may be associated with weakness and loss of sensation. Vitamin B_{12} stores normally fall in older people, and deficiency should always be considered with those developing dementia.

Care must be taken to differentiate megaloblastic anaemia from myelodysplastic syndrome, which may be associated with a refractory macrocytic anaemia. Serum concentrations of vitamin B_{12}, folate, and red cell folate should be measured, and occasionally a bone marrow examination may be indicated.

The importance of identifying any deficiency anaemia is that, although the effects may be relatively mild initially, they can progress and severely incapacitate a previously active pensioner. The deficiencies can be easily reversed, and supplements should be continued for as long as the underlying problem remains.

Anaemia of chronic disease

Any prolonged illness such as infection, malignant disease, renal disease, or connective tissue disorder may be accompanied by a moderate fall in the haemoglobin concentration. This seldom drops below 90-100 g/l and is typically normocytic and normochromic. Haematinics will not increase the haemoglobin concentration, which may improve only after treatment of the underlying condition. This condition may not always be apparent, and a general screen may be needed for underlying malignancy or systemic disease.

Malignancies

Most forms of malignancy are more common in elderly people than in the rest of the population. The myelodysplastic syndromes and chronic lymphocytic leukaemia are frequently found incidentally, and their diagnosis does not necessarily indicate the need for treatment. Each patient must be considered individually so that the possible benefits of treatment can be balanced against side effects and considered in the light of any improvement in the quality of life.

The graph is adapted with permission from Newland *et al* (*N Engl J Med* 1984;310: 261-2).

Further reading

- Hann IM, Gibson BES, Letsky EA, eds. *Fetal and neonatal haematology*. London: Baillière Tindall, 1991.
- Lilleyman JS, Hann IM, eds. *Pediatric hematology*. New York: Churchill Livingstone, 1992.

14 HAEMATOLOGICAL EMERGENCIES

Rebecca Frewin, Andrew Henson, Drew Provan

> General physicians must be able to recognise and start basic treatment, which may be life saving, in patients presenting with haematological emergencies

Patients with both malignant and non-malignant haematological disease may present with dramatic and often life threatening complications of their diseases. This article deals with five of the most common emergencies encountered by haematologists. Although these conditions are not seen commonly in day to day clinical practice, recognition of the underlying pathological processes is important in determining the likely cause of the abnormalities and is helpful in determining the specific treatment needed.

Hyperviscosity syndrome

Causes of hyperviscosity

- Myeloma (especially IgA)
- Waldenström's macroglobulinaemia (IgM paraprotein)
- Polycythaemia
- High white cell count (hyperleucocytosis)

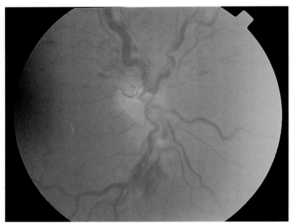

Figure 14.1 Fundal changes in patient with hyperviscosity (newly diagnosed myeloma with IgA concentration of 50 g/l).

This may be caused by several haematological conditions. Blood viscosity is a function of the concentration and composition of its components. A marked increase in plasma proteins (for example, monoclonal immunoglobulin in myeloma) or cellular constituents (for example, white blood cells in acute leukaemia) will raise the overall blood viscosity. This leads to sludging of the microcirculation and a variety of clinical manifestations. Hyperviscosity may present insidiously or acutely with neurological symptoms and signs.

Blood viscosity will often be more than four times the normal viscosity before symptoms occur. Patients with chronic disorders such as polycythaemia and myeloma are often physiologically well compensated for the degree of hyperviscosity and may complain only of mild headaches. In contrast, patients with acute leukaemia and a high white cell count may present in extremis; they become hypoxic from pulmonary involvement and are often obtunded, with a variety of neurological signs. Prompt treatment is needed to prevent permanent deficits. Elderly patients with impaired left ventricular function may experience decompensation due to their hyperviscosity, resulting in increasing congestive cardiac failure.

Symptoms and signs of hyperviscosity

- Mild headache
- Neurological disturbance
    - Ataxia
    - Nystagmus
    - Vertigo
    - Confusion
    - Changes in mental state
    - Coma
- Visual disturbance
    - Blurring of vision
    - Dilatation and segmentation of retinal veins
    - "Sausage" appearance of retinal veins
    - Risk of central retinal vein occlusion
- Genitourinary or gastrointestinal bleeding

Symptoms occur when the viscosity of the blood is more than four times that of water

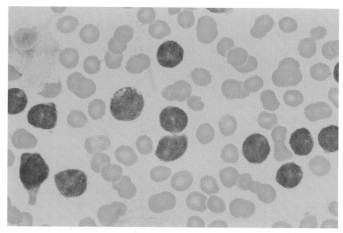

Figure 14.2 Blood film in patient with hyperviscosity due to hyperleucocytosis (4 year old child with newly diagnosed acute lymphoblastic leukaemia (white cell count 200×10⁹/l)).

> Plasmapheresis may be used both for acute attacks and long term—for example, as palliative treatment for patients resistant to, or unable to tolerate, chemotherapy

The definitive treatment of patients with hyperviscosity is dependent on the underlying pathology. For patients presenting with acute leukaemia, vigorous intravenous hydration and intensive chemotherapy often results in a rapid reduction in the white cell count. Leukapheresis may be used as an interim measure until chemotherapy exerts its full effect. For patients with myeloma or Waldenström's macroglobulinaemia (a low grade lymphoma characterised by production of monoclonal IgM, most of which is intravascular) plasmapheresis effectively reduces the paraprotein concentration.

Sickle cell crisis

Sickle cell crises

Vaso-occlusive—In any tissue but especially bones, chest, and abdomen (eg splenic infarcts); in cerebral vessels, leading to stroke
Aplastic—In parvovirus B19 infection
Sequestration—Particularly in infants and young children; massive pooling of red cells in spleen and other organs, leading to precipitous drop in haemoglobin
Haemolytic—Further reduction in life span of red cells, leading to worsening anaemia and features of haemolysis
Chest syndrome—Pleuritic pain and fever may mimic pneumonia or pulmonary embolism; progressive respiratory failure

Treatment of sickle cell crises

- Vigorous intravenous hydration
- Adequate analgesia—for example, intravenous opiates
- Broad spectrum antibiotics
- Oxygen therapy
- Consider exchange blood transfusion

The sickling disorders (Hb SS, Hb SC, Hb S/β thalassaemia, and Hb SD) are inherited structural haemoglobin variants. Homozygous Hb SS in particular is associated with several complications, including recurrent vaso-occlusive crises, leg ulcers, renal impairment, hyposplenism, and retinopathy.

Sickle cell crises include vaso-occlusive, aplastic, sequestration, and haemolytic episodes. The chest syndrome and the girdle syndrome are more severe forms of crisis associated with higher morbidity and mortality.

Crises may be precipitated by dehydration or infection; in many cases no obvious precipitant is found.

The aim of treatment is to break the vicious cycle of sickling: sickling results in hypoxia and acidosis, which in turn precipitate further sickling. This is exacerbated by dehydration, and a high fluid intake (70 ml/kg/24 h) is the cornerstone of management.

Also imperative in managing sickle cell crises is adequate pain relief—opiates, by continuous subcutaneous or intravenous infusions, may be needed. Arterial blood gas pressures should be performed and oxygen therapy prescribed if hypoxia is confirmed. It should be remembered that sickle cell patients are functionally asplenic and that infection is a common precipitant of crises. Broad spectrum antibiotics should be started while waiting for the results of blood and urine cultures.

It is important to recognise the patients who need urgent exchange transfusion to reduce the level of Hb S to below 30%. Transfusion should be started promptly if the patient has a severe chest syndrome (with pronounced hypoxia), has had a cardiovascular accident, or has priapism.

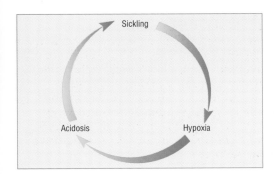

Figure 14.3 Vicious cycle in sickle cell crisis.

Spinal cord compression

Symptoms and signs of cord compression

- Back pain
- Weakness in legs
- Upper motor neurone and sensory signs
- Loss of sphincter control (bowels/bladder)

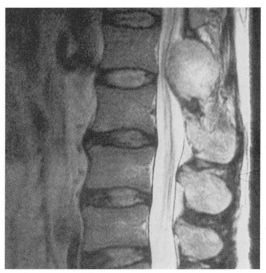

Figure 14.4 Magnetic resonance image showing spinal cord compression.

Neurosurgical advice should be obtained as in some cases surgical decompression may allow recovery of function

---

Some patients may present at the haematology clinic with metastatic tumour deposits—for example, lymphoma or plasmacytoma—resulting in cord compression. Commonly, overt cord compression is preceded by signs consistent with root compression, with pain in the affected dermatome. Most patients with cord compression complain of pain—it is often constant and easily confused with that of pain due to degenerative disease. Often it is not until more overt neurological signs are manifested that a diagnosis of cord compression is considered.

The neurological signs accompanying cord compression vary according to both the rapidity of development of compression and the area of cord affected. Acute lesions often result in hypotonia and weakness, whereas chronic lesions are more often associated with the classic upper motor neurone signs of hypertonia and hyper-reflexia. The associated sensory loss is defined by the site of the lesion, but hyperaesthesia may be seen in the dermatome at the level of the lesion. More lateral lesions may result in a dissociative sensory loss—that is, ipsilateral loss of joint position sense and proprioception with contralateral loss of pain and temperature. Bladder and bowel disturbances often occur late, with the exception of the cauda equina compression syndrome, in which they are an early feature.

If cord compression is suspected the patient should be investigated with plain spinal radiography, which may show evidence of lytic lesions (as, for example, in myeloma). The definitive investigation is magnetic resonance imaging to delineate the level of the lesion and to help plan further treatment.

In a patient presenting de novo with cord compression further investigations (protein electrophoresis, measurement of prostatic specific antigen and other tumour markers, and chest radiography) are needed to elucidate the underlying cause. A formal biopsy of the lesion may be needed to determine the underlying pathology.

In an acute presentation high dose dexamethasone (for example, 4 mg four times daily) is given. Further management depends on the underlying cause, but often a combination of chemotherapy and radiotherapy is given.

Disseminated intravascular coagulation

Clinical features of disseminated intravascular coagulation

Bleeding
- Spontaneous bruising
- Petechiae
- Prolonged bleeding from venepuncture sites, arterial lines, etc
- Bleeding into gastrointestinal tract or lungs
- Secondary bleeding after surgery
- Coma (intracerebral bleeding)

Clotting
- Acute renal failure (ischaemia of renal cortex)
- Venous thromboembolism
- Skin necrosis or gangrene
- Liver failure (due to infection and hypotension)
- Coma (cerebral infarction)

Shock
- Due to underlying disease together with disseminated intravascular coagulation

Central nervous system
- Transient neurological symptoms and signs
- Coma
- Delirium

Lungs
- Transient hypoxaemia
- Pulmonary haemorrhage
- Adult respiratory distress syndrome

Disseminated intravascular coagulation describes the syndrome of widespread intravascular coagulation induced by blood procoagulants either introduced into or produced in the bloodstream. These coagulant proteins overcome the normal physiological anticoagulant mechanisms. The overall result, irrespective of cause, is widespread tissue ischaemia (due to clot formation, thrombi) and bleeding (due to consumption of clotting factors, platelets, and the production of breakdown products that further inhibit the coagulation pathway).

The diagnosis of disseminated intravascular coagulation is initially clinical and is confirmed by various blood tests. There are many causes of disseminated intravascular coagulation, including obstetric emergencies, infections, neoplasms, trauma, and vascular disorders.

Main investigations* for disseminated intravascular coagulation

Investigation	Positive result
Full blood count	Decreased platelet count
Prothrombin time	Increased
Activated partial thromboplastin time	Increased
Fibrinogen	Decreased
Fibrin degradation products/D dimers	Increased

* Other investigations: urea and electrolytes, liver function tests, blood cultures, pulse oximetry (oxygen saturation)

Causes of acute disseminated intravascular coagulation

Infection—Especially Gram negative infections, endotoxic shock
Obstetric—Placental abruption, intrauterine fetal death, severe pre-eclampsia or eclampsia, amniotic fluid embolism
Trauma—Especially head injury, burns
Malignancy—Carcinoma of prostate, lung, pancreas, ovary, and gastrointestinal tract
Miscellaneous—Transfusion with incompatible blood group, drug reactions, hypothermia, venomous snake bite, transplant rejection
Vascular—Aortic aneurysm, giant haemangioma

Initial management of disseminated intravascular coagulation

- Treat as for severe bleeding/shock
- Establish intravenous access (large bore cannula)
- Restore circulating volume—with, for example, crystalloids
- Administer fresh frozen plasma and cryoprecipitate and regularly monitor full blood count, prothrombin time, and activated partial thromboplastin time
- Consider giving platelet transfusion
- Remove the underlying cause

Treatment is primarily directed at the underlying cause—for example, the use of antibiotics when infection is suspected, or removal of fetus and placenta with placental abruption or retained dead fetus syndrome. Disseminated intravascular coagulation generally resolves fairly quickly after removal of the underlying cause.

Interim supportive measures, such as intravenous hydration and oxygen therapy, are important. Correction of the coagulopathy entails the use of fresh frozen plasma, cryoprecipitate, and platelet transfusion. No uniform protocol exists for transfusing blood and blood products. Instead, for each patient the quantity of blood product used is decided after clinical evaluation and serial coagulation assays.

The use of intravenous heparin to treat disseminated intravascular coagulation remains controversial. Some evidence supports the value of heparin in the management of acute promyelocytic leukaemia, the dead fetus syndrome, and aortic aneurysm before resection. For other causes of disseminated intravascular coagulation the use of heparin is more uncertain and may actually worsen the bleeding.

Infection in patients with impaired immunity

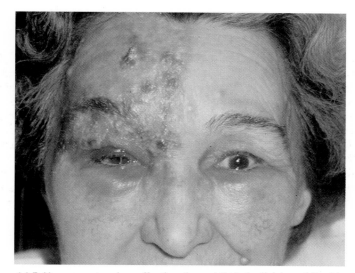

Figure 14.5 Herpes zoster virus affecting the ophthalmic division of the trigeminal nerve in patient with chronic lymphocytic leukaemia.

Patients with a variety of haematological diseases are immunocompromised due to either their underlying disease or the treatment required for the condition. For example, patients with myeloma often present with recurrent infection as a result of the reduction in normal immunoglobulin concentrations associated with the paraproteinaemia. This susceptibility is compounded by the use of combination chemotherapy, which may render them neutropenic.

Several haematological disorders are now routinely treated in outpatient clinics with aggressive chemotherapy, so some patients in the community may be neutropenic as a result of this. Patients are educated to seek medical advice immediately if they develop any infection since Gram negative septicaemia may lead rapidly to death. For patients receiving intensive chemotherapy presenting with fever while neutropenic, broad spectrum antibiotics should be started immediately. The choice of antibiotics depends on local microbiological advice in the light of the sensitivities of the micro-organisms in the region.

Risks of infection in patients with no spleen or hypofunctioning spleen

- With encapsulated organisms—for example, *Streptococcus pneumoniae* (60%), *Haemophilus influenzae* type b, *Neisseria meningitidis*
- Less commonly—*Escherichia coli*, malaria, babesiosis, *Capnocytophaga canimorsus*

Recommendations for patients with no spleen or hypofunctioning spleen*

- Pneumococcal vaccine (Pneumovax II) 0.5 ml— two weeks before splenectomy or as soon as possible after splenectomy (for example, if emergency splenectomy is performed); reimmunise every 5-10 years
- *H influenzae* type b (Hib) vaccine 0.5 ml
- Meningococcal polysaccharide vaccine for *N meningitidis* type A and C 0.5 ml
- Penicillin as prophylaxis (250 mg twice daily—for life)

The three vaccines (subcutaneous or intramuscular) may be given at same time, but different sites should be used
* Based on the guidelines for the prevention and treatment of infection in patients with an absent or dysfunctional spleen, *BMJ* 1996;312:430-4

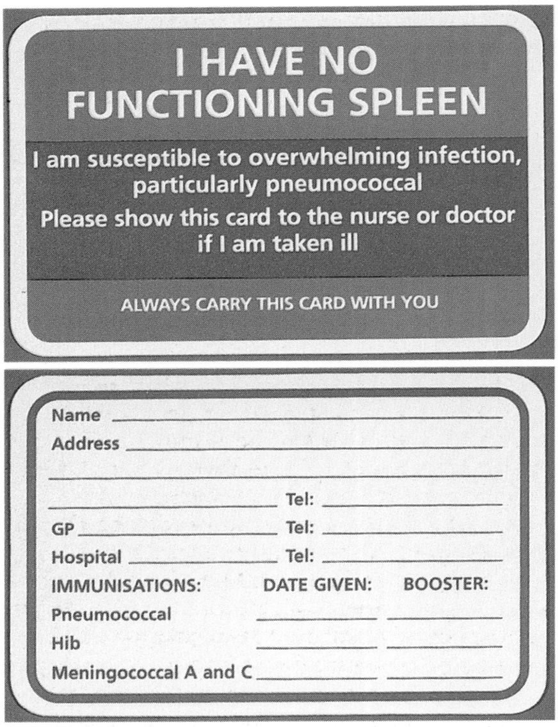

I HAVE NO FUNCTIONING SPLEEN

I am susceptible to overwhelming infection, particularly pneumococcal

Please show this card to the nurse or doctor if I am taken ill

ALWAYS CARRY THIS CARD WITH YOU

Name _____
Address _____
_____
_____ Tel: _____
GP _____ Tel: _____
Hospital _____ Tel: _____

IMMUNISATIONS:	DATE GIVEN:	BOOSTER:
Pneumococcal		
Hib		
Meningococcal A and C		

Figure 14.6 Card carried by patients with no spleen or hypofunctioning spleen.

Patients with chronic lymphocytic leukaemia often have recurrent infection in the absence of neutropenia, because of the accompanying hypogammaglobulinaemia seen in this disorder. Frequent courses of antibiotics are often required. The role of regular intravenous immunoglobulin infusions to "boost" their immunity is debatable. Patients with chronic lymphocytic leukaemia may develop severe recurrent herpes zoster infections. Prompt treatment with aciclovir should always be given at the first suspicion of any herpetic lesions developing, and hospital referral for intravenous antibiotics and aciclovir should be considered if the lesions are not confined to a single dermatome or are in a delicate area—for example, ophthalmic division of trigeminal nerve.

Patients who are functionally or anatomically asplenic are at high risk of infection with encapsulated organisms, especially Streptococcus pneumoniae.

Penicillin prophylaxis and immunisation reduces the incidence of these infections but does not abolish the risk completely. If any of these patients becomes acutely unwell the prompt administration of 1200 mg benzylpenicillin (if no history of allergy to penicillin) and prompt referral for further treatment may be life saving.

Dr Ken Tung, consultant radiologist, Southampton University Hospitals Trust, provided the magnetic resonance image. The photograph showing herpes zoster virus is published with permission from *Clinical Haematology— a Postgraduate Exam Companion* (Provan D, Amos TA, Smith AG, Oxford: Butterworth-Heinemann, 1997).

15 THE FUTURE OF HAEMATOLOGY, MOLECULAR BIOLOGY, AND GENE THERAPY

Adele K Fielding, Sally Ager, Stephen J Russell

The future of haematology–diagnosis and treatment

Diagnosis
- Increasing automation giving quicker and more reliable results—eg automated cross matching; automated diagnostic polymerase chain reaction
- More DNA/RNA based diagnosis, allowing increased diagnostic precision—eg precise definition of genetic abnormalities; diagnosis with polymerase chain reaction
- More "near patient" testing, allowing rapid screening—eg haemoglobinometers, monitoring of anticoagulant treatment

Treatment
- New drugs—eg tailored to molecular abnormalities
- New biological agents—eg thrombopoietin, which may speed platelet recovery after chemotherapy
- Transplantation across tissue barriers—eg cord blood transplantation
- Blood substitutes—eg recombinant haemoglobin
- Gene therapy—probably for many haematological disorders

This article will assess the impact of advances in science and technology on the practice of haematology and attempt to predict how haematology will change further over the next 10 to 15 years.

The major advances in scientific thought and technological development that have already changed the practice of modern haematology are likely to affect both laboratory diagnosis and treatment in the future. This article will address three specific area of haematology—anaemia, haemophilia, and leukaemia—and explain how important innovations could be expected to change clinical practice in these areas. The article begins, however, with an overview of gene therapy, which, although currently some way from curing haematological diseases, is likely to have a role in most areas of haematological practice in the future.

Both diagnostically and therapeutically, the identification of the molecular pathology of the underlying disorder will continue to steer the future, but the ability to make more accurate diagnoses has not yet resulted in improved treatment.

Gene therapy

Gene therapy strategies

Strategy	Potential application
Corrective replacement	Sickle cell disease—to replace the point mutation that causes the substitution of valine for glutamine on the sixth amino acid residue of the β globin chain
Corrective gene addition	Haemophilia—to introduce a gene for missing coagulation protein
Corrective antisense treatment	Low grade non-Hodgkin's lymphoma (NHL)—to introduce antisense oligonucleotides, preventing BCL2 overexpression, which is responsible for the failure of the lymphoma cells to undergo apoptosis
Pharmacological	Continuous production of interferon alfa, erythropoietin, or other therapeutic proteins
Cytotoxic	Leukaemia—targeted delivery of cytotoxic proteins
Prophylactic	Chemoprotection—drug resistance genes introduced into haemopoietic stem cells, conferring resistant phenotype, thus protecting against chemotherapeutic agents
Immunostimulatory	Idiotypic vaccination—in B cell tumours such as NHL and myeloma the variable region sequences of the surface immunoglobulin of the tumour cell provide a tumour specific antigen against which an individualised vaccine for each patient can be produced

The term gene therapy is applied to any manoeuvre in which genes or genetically modified cells are introduced into a patient for therapeutic benefit. Gene therapy is still in its infancy, and despite the potential of the approach, clinical benefit has yet to be shown.

Successful gene therapy depends on the availability of reliable methods for delivering a gene into the nuclei of selected target cells and subsequently ensuring the regulation of gene expression. Haematological cells are readily accessible for manipulation and so can be genetically modified outside the body and reinfused. The aim in the future, however, will be to modify the target cells without first removing them from the patient. Genes that are to be delivered to cells must first be inserted into plasmids. These small circular molecules of double stranded DNA derived from bacteria can then be used to transfer therapeutic genes to cells by physical methods or by insertion into recombinant viruses.

Whichever vector system is used, the barriers through which the therapeutic genes must be transported to reach their destination are the same. Many viral and non-viral vector systems are being developed to try to achieve the steps outlined here, and it is often difficult to choose the most appropriate vector for a particular application.

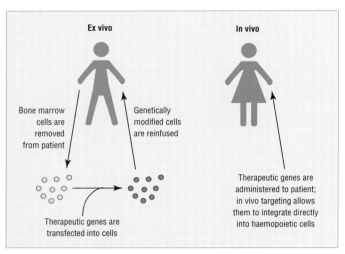

Figure 15.1   Ex vivo and in vivo gene transfer strategies.

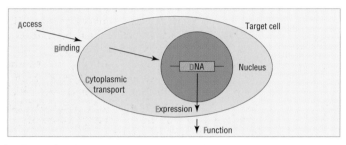

Figure 15.2 ABC of gene therapy—A vector must be able to access the cells to be transduced and bind to and penetrate the membrane of the target cell. Once inside the nucleus, the exogenous DNA must be integrated into the cellular genome if stable expression is required. Gene expression must be at a high enough level and sufficiently regulated for clinical benefit.

For gene therapy applications, where it is crucial to achieve gene expression in the progeny of the target (modified) cells, it is important to use a vector that stably inserts its genes into the chromosome of the host cell, and retrovirus vectors are the most suitable for this purpose. For direct in vivo gene delivery, vector attachment to a specific target cell is a vital additional requirement. Such vector targeting is at last beginning to look like a realistic possibility.

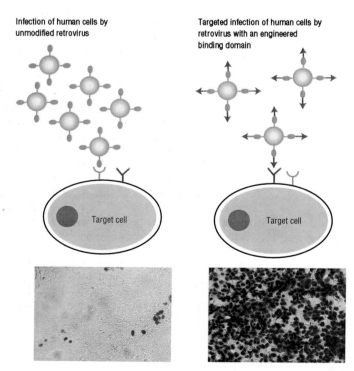

Figure 15.3 Retroviral vectors used for gene therapy usually infect cells via a naturally occurring receptor on the surface of human cells. They can, however, be engineered to display on their surface various ligands that are capable of binding to their specific receptors on target cells. In vitro, infection can be shown by X gal staining (successfully infected cells turn blue).

Anaemia

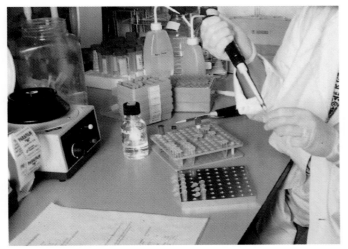

Figure 15.4 Polymerase chain reaction can be carried out with a minimum of specialist equipment.

Prenatal options from diagnosis based on polymerase chain reaction

Tissue used	Strategies permitted
Chorionic villus	Selective termination of affected fetus; in utero organ transplantation; in utero gene therapy
Polar body	Gamete selection (egg only, for in vitro fertilisation)
6-8 Cell embryo (after in vitro fertilisation)	Embryo selection
Blastocyst (after in vitro fertilisation)	Embryo selection

Requirements for the production of recombinant haemoglobin

- A source of protoporphyrin IX (haem)—this prosthetic group is common to haem containing protein of many species and thus can be produced endogenously
- Synthesis of α and β globins
- A method of production that is suitable for large scale production and purification. This may be in microbial or mammalian cells or in transgenic animals. The former may result in structural and functional alterations as a result of expressing the proteins in bacteria or yeast

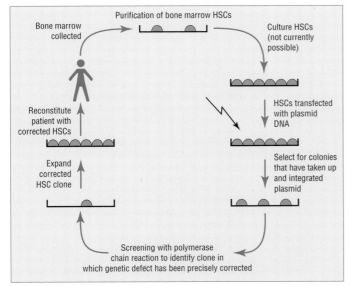

Figure 15.5 Stem cell surgery. Ideally, haemopoietic stem cells would be isolated from the bone marrow, followed by expansion of haemopoietic stem cells (HSCs) before purified cells are grown in culture and transfected with the DNA to correct the defect. The plasmid carrying the therapeutic DNA also carries a selectable marker (for example, an antibiotic resistance gene), which would allow colonies that contain the successfully integrated DNA to be selected.

The move away from the main laboratory towards units nearer to patients—such as intensive care units, general practice surgeries—is likely to provide rapid and increasingly reliable testing of basic haematological variables outside the formal laboratory environment. A large haematology laboratory providing a centralised quality assured service will still be required, but along with the automated analysers, diagnostic tests based on polymerase chain reaction will be used increasingly.

With the identification of the precise mutations associated with many forms of hereditary anaemias, routine characterisation by nucleic acid sequence analysis will facilitate the use of disease specific diagnostic tests based on polymerase chain reaction. This will provide more precise prognostic information for affected individuals as well as accurate identification of affected embryos. As reliable prenatal diagnosis at an early stage will be available, so will an increasing range of prenatal treatment options.

For patients affected by hereditary anaemias such as sickle cell disease and thalassaemia, advances in transplantation immunology may permit transplantation across tissue barriers, making bone marrow transplantation a treatment option for all affected patients. In addition, gene therapy for these disorders could provide another potentially curative strategy, although the genetic correction of hereditary anaemias still presents complex challenges. In sickle cell disease, for example, delivery of normal copies of the β globin gene to haemopoietic stem cells will be insufficient for cure. As continued Hb S production would be damaging, the mutated β globin genes must also be removed. Stem cell surgery techniques might be used to achieve such an aim.

Fully automated crossmatching procedures will soon be in place in all haematology laboratories, but in the longer term, genetically engineered recombinant haemoglobin is likely to replace transfusion with blood derived from donors. The use of artificial haemoglobin solutions has been associated with various toxicities including renal toxicity due to the renal filtration of haemoglobin dimers. Production of modified recombinant haemoglobin or in vitro modification of a recombinant product will hopefully overcome this problem.

Haemophilia

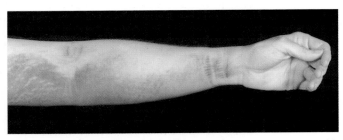

Figure 15.6 Haemophilic patient with inhibitors and severe spontaneous bleeding. Currently the development of inhibitors represents one of the biggest problems facing patients with haemophilia.

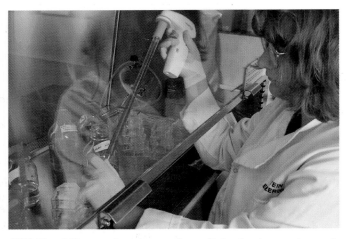

Figure 15.7 The ability to culture mammalian cells in vitro has made a major contribution to research in many areas of modern haematology.

As specific mutations have now been identified to account for a large proportion of patients with haemophilia, routine characterisation of all haemophilias by direct sequence analysis is likely. This will facilitate accurate carrier diagnosis and thus the use of disease specific diagnostic tests based on polymerase chain reaction for accurate identification of affected embryos. As for the inherited anaemias, several prenatal treatments are likely to become available.

Dependence on blood products with the attendant risk of viral transmission has been disastrous for many patients with haemophilia but is unlikely to be a problem in the future. Recombinant human factor VIII is already available, recombinant coagulation factor VIIa is improving the prospects for haemophilic patients with inhibitors to factor VIII, and the development of other recombinant coagulation factors will ultimately obviate the need to use fractionated human blood. Definitive gene therapy of haemophilia also has excellent prospects. Haemophilia is known to be curable by liver transplantation, indicating that it should also be curable by genetic modification of host cells to produce normal factor VIII. Regulation of gene expression is not thought to be a critical issue as a moderate excess of factor VIII has no known procoagulant effect. There are concerns that cells producing factor VIII might be recognised as "foreign" by the patient and rejected. A solution to this type of problem may lie in the recent demonstration that the rejection of foreign cells can be prevented when they are genetically modified to express Fas ligand, which triggers apoptotic cell death of cytotoxic T cells that enter the graft before they can cause any damage.

Leukaemia

An understanding of the molecular mechanism of malignant transformation in leukaemia forms the basis for improved diagnostic sensitivity and the monitoring of minimal residual disease and paves the way for more directed treatment interventions, including the eventual possibility of targeting the causative genetic defects. Assays based on polymerase chain reaction, which can detect one malignant cell in a population of 10^5 cells, are a highly sensitive diagnostic and monitoring tool, and the full implications of detection of minimal residual disease at various times during the treatment of leukaemia are not yet known. Assays based on polymerase chain reaction will also be used in conjunction with powerful immunophenotyping methods (that is, monoclonal antibodies capable of detecting specific cell surface molecules on malignant cells) to follow the fates of individual neoplastic subpopulations in response to different types of treatment.

In the treatment of acute leukaemia dose intensification with stem cell support seems to confer some benefit for patients—but at the expense of increased toxicity, so that overall survival seems not to have been improved by high dose strategies with autologous transplantation. So far, the use of blood rather than bone marrow as a source of

Scientific techniques and approaches that have made major contributions to modern haematology

Technique	Applications in haematology
Gene cloning and sequencing allow identification, characterisation, and manipulation of genes responsible for specific products or diseases	• Elucidation of the molecular pathology of disease and diagnostic tests based on the polymerase chain reaction
Polymerase chain reaction is a highly sensitive and versatile technique for amplifying very small quantities of DNA. Amplification of RNA molecules is possible after initial reverse transcription of RNA into DNA (RT-PCR)	• Rapid diagnosis of infectious diseases in immunocompromised patients (for example, hepatitis C); minimal residual disease detection in haematological malignancies where the molecular defect is known; carrier detection and antenatal diagnosis in haemophilias and hereditary anaemias
Monoclonal antibodies allow immunohistochemistry of tissue and cells, analysis and cell sorting with fluorescence activated cell sorter (FACS), and cell purification	• Increased diagnostic precision, "positive purging," ex vivo gene delivery, and ex vivo expansion of progenitor cells are possible as a result of the fact that populations of haemopoietic cells containing a high proportion of primitive progenitors can be isolated
Mammalian tissue culture and gene transfer to mammalian cells provide methods for studying gene expression. Reporter genes can be used to study gene expression in cell lines in vitro. Transgenic animals can be created by inserting intact or manipulated genes into the germ line of an animal providing an in vivo model of gene function	• Allows gene therapy, tissue engineering, and study of gene expression and function
Protein engineering and construction of recombinant proteins allow production of large quantities of human proteins. Proteins with modified or novel functions can be rationally designed and produced	• Recombinant drugs (for example, the haemopoietic growth factors), antibody engineering to produce therapeutic antibodies, recombinant blood products free from risk of viral contamination

Glossary

General molecular biology
• Recombinant DNA—Any DNA sequence that does not occur naturally but is formed by joining DNA segments from different sources
• Polymerase chain reaction—Process by which genes or gene segments can be rapidly, conveniently, and accurately copied, producing up to 10^{12} copies of the original sequence in a few hours
• Reverse transcription—Process by which RNA is used as a template for the production of a DNA copy
• Transcription factor-Protein that is able to bind to chromosomal DNA close to a gene and thereby regulates the expression of the gene

Haematology and immunology
• Stem cell—Pluripotent cell that has the ability to renew itself or differentiate. The haemopoietic stem cell gives rise to all lineages of haemopoietic cells
• Minimal residual disease—Cancer that is still present in the body after treatment but remains undetectable by conventional means—for example, light microscopy
• Immunophenotype—The cell surface markers on any given cell detected by the use of monoclonal antibodies
• Chromosome translocations—Areas of chromosomes may break and rejoin with other chromosomes (for example, t(8;21), where an area of chromosome 8 is abnormally fused to an area of chromosome 21) or break off and rejoin "back to front" (for example, inv16)
• Fas ligand—The ligand that binds to the cell surface molecule Fas (CD95) which is normally found on the surface of lymphocytes. When Fas ligand binds to its receptor, cell death (apoptosis) is triggered
• Apoptosis—Programmed cell death
• Adoptive immunotherapy—The transfer of immune cells for therapeutic benefit
• Transgenic animals—Animals with an intact or manipulated gene inserted into their germline

haemopoietic stem cells, despite its advantages of faster haemopoietic recovery and economy, has not influenced treatment related mortality. It is possible that new haemopoietic growth factors, such as thrombopoietin, may speed engraftment sufficiently to have a beneficial effect. Although the freezer provides chemoprotection for haemopoietic stem cells, other normal tissues cannot be protected in this way, and methods for reducing extramedullary toxicity are likely to be developed.

The delineation of molecular defects should finally allow a more subtle approach towards the treatment of leukaemia. For example, it is already known that acute myeloid leukaemias associated with specific chromosomal rearrangements—such as inversion of chromosome 16, inv(16), or translocation of DNA between chromosomes 8 and 21, t(8;21)—are associated with a good prognosis and that their respective chromosomal translocations involve the opposite halves of a single heterodimeric transcription factor. Studies on the t(15;17) translocation in acute promyelocytic leukaemia pointed to deregulated expression of the translocated retinoic acid receptor gene as a retrospective explanation for the efficacy of retinoic acid in this disease, and new drugs directed at therapeutic targets such as the heterodimeric transcription factor described above are now likely to be developed.

Gene therapy strategies are also possible for leukaemia. Already the transfer of drug resistance genes as chemoprotection for normal haemopoietic stem cells during chemotherapy is being investigated clinically. Many other strategies are possible, such as the targeted delivery of cytotoxic proteins and the use of adoptive immunotherapy with genetically modified T cells.

INDEX

abdominal distension 25
abdominal mass 47
abdominal pain 54
ablative therapy 51, 53
achlorhydria 5
aciclovir 55, 64
acidosis 61
acoustic nerve damage 13
activated partial thromboplastin time 43, 63
activated protein C resistance 45
acute leukaemia 24–8
    classification 24
    incidence 25
    investigations 26
    management 26–7
    predisposing factors 24
    presentation 25
    toxicity of treatments 26
acute lymphoblastic leukaemia 24–5, 52
acute myeloid leukaemia 24–5, 52
    myelodysplastic syndrome 34
acute promyelocytic leukaemia 63, 69
acute tumour lysis syndrome 49
Addison's disease 5
adoptive immunotherapy 69
adriamycin 42
AIDS related non-Hodgkin's lymphoma 50
air filtration 54
alcohol 5, 7, 17, 30, 43
alkaline phosphatase 21, 40
alkylating agents 24, 34, 48
alloantibodies 58
allogeneic bone marrow transplantation 22, 27,
        37, 41, 51–3
    see also bone marrow transplantation
allopurinol 27
all-trans-retinoic acid (ATRA) 27
alopecia 54
Alport's syndrome 30
amegakaryocytic thrombocytopenia 29
amniotic fluid embolism 63
amyloidosis 39–41, 44
anaemia 24, 34, 40, 42, 43, 47
    aplastic 5, 7–8, 26, 30, 52
    Blackfan-Diamond 15
    of chronic disease 59
    congenital dyserythropoetic 15
    future of treatment 67–8
    haemolytic 9, 10–15, 56
    hereditary 10–15, 67
    hypochromic 1–4, 12
    infection 56–7
    iron deficiency 1–4, 58–9
    macrocytic 5–9, 34, 59
    megaloblastic 6, 59
    microcytic 1–4
    neonatal 56
    normochromic normocytic 40, 56, 59
    pernicious 5–8, 59
    refractory 36
    sickle cell see sickle cell disease
    sideroblastic 2–3
    thalassaemia see thalassaemia
anagrelide 19
analgesia 41
ancrod 33
anencephaly 6

angina 59
angular stomatitis 1
ankylosing spondylitis 20
Ann Arbor staging 47, 50
antibiotic resistance gene 67
antibiotics 11–12, 37, 41, 48, 61, 64
    prophylactic 54–5
antibody engineering 69
antibody therapy (targeted) 48
anticoagulation 32–3, 45–6
anticonvulsant drugs 58
anti-D immunoglobulin 56
anti-endomysial antibodies 8
antifungal agents 54
antigen 48
antigliadin antibodies 8
antimalarials 12, 14
antiphospholipid (lupus) syndrome 30, 45
antiplatelet antibodies 58
antireticulin antibodies 8
antisene oligonucleotides 65
antithrombin deficiency 45
Anthony Nolan bone marrow registry 52
aortic aneurysm 63
aplastic anaemia 5, 7–8, 26, 30, 52
aplastic crisis 11, 57
arterial blood gases 61
arterial obstruction 7
arterial thrombosis 45
arthralgia 4
arthritis 13
arthropathy 44
ascorbic acid 1
aseptic necrosis 11–12
aspergillus 54
asphyxia 58
aspirin 19, 31–3, 43, 45, 59
asplenism 61, 64
ataxia 60
ataxia telangiectasia 24
atherosclerosis 45
ATRA (all-trans-retinoic acid) 27
atrophic gastritis 8
autoantibodies 8, 30, 44
autoimmune disease 48, 52, 55
autoimmune gastritis 5, 48
autologous stem cell transplantation 22, 41,
        51–3
    see also bone marrow transplantation
azathioprine 7, 33

BACUP (British Association of Cancer United
        Patients) 21
BCR-ABL gene 20–1
Bence Jones protein 39–40
benzene 24
benzylpenicillin 64
Bernard-Soulier syndrome 30
bilirubin 6
Binet staging 47
biphosphonate therapy 41
Blackfan-Diamond anaemia 15
blast cells 26
blast crisis 20, 23
bleeding, abnormal 2, 25, 32, 34, 43–5, 56–9, 62
bleeding disorders 16, 19, 25, 31, 43–5, 57

bleeding time 43
blindness 11
blood crossmatching 67
blood group 5
blood product support 32
blood stasis 45
blood transfusion 4, 12, 13, 19, 26
    exchange 58, 61
Bloom's syndrome 24
bone destruction 39
bone marrow aspiration 3, 8, 18, 29, 21, 26, 34
    abnormal plasma cells 40
bone marrow biopsy 47
bone marrow changes 5, 13, 34
bone marrow chromosomal analysis 17
bone marrow failure 24–8, 32–3, 34, 36
bone marrow fibrosis 19
bone marrow harvest 52–3
bone marrow registries 52
bone marrow transplantation 13, 24, 27, 29, 30,
        51–5
    allogeneic 37, 41, 52–3
    autologous 22, 41, 52–3
    complications 54
    costs 55
    definition 51
    graft versus host disease 54
    future developments 55, 67
    history 51
    procedures 53
bone marrow trephine 18, 19, 34
bone pain 11–12, 23, 25, 39–41
bone rarefaction 40
brain syndrome 11–12
breast cancer 52
breast feeding 4, 58
bruising 25, 34, 43–4, 58, 62
    see also ecchymoses
buccal desquamation 54
Burkitt's lymphoma 49
busulphan 17, 19, 21, 23

candida 54
cardiac failure 2, 6, 19, 42, 60
cardiolipin antibodies 45
cardiovascular disease 7
carmustine 42
cataracts 28, 54
cauda equina compression syndrome 62
cell purification 69
cell separation 51, 52–3
central nervous system impairment 40
cerebrospinal prophylaxis 49
chemoprotection 65, 69
chemoradiotherapy 51–4
chest infections 54
chest syndrome 61
chlorambucil 34, 42, 48
chorionic villus sampling 13, 67
Christmas disease 57
chromosomal fragility 29
chromosomal translocation 69
chromosome analysis 35
chronic lymphocytic leukaemia 39, 42, 47–8, 63
    Binet staging 47
chronic myeloid leukaemia 20–3, 52, 69

Index

acute phase 23
  blast crisis 20, 23
  chronic phase 21–2
  pathogenesis 20
chronic myelomonocytic leukaemia 35, 37
cirrhosis 44
cleft palate 6
clinical trials 24
  see also Medical Research Council trials
clonal disorders 16–19, 20–3, 24–8, 34
clotting *see* coagulation
coagulation 29, 62
  factors 29, 43–4, 46
  screening 26
coagulation factor concentrate 46
coagulation factor deficiency 43–4
cobalamin *see* vitamin B12
coeliac disease 2
collagen 29
collagen vascular disorder 45
colorectal cancer 3
coma 60, 62
computed tomography 47
confusion 60
congenital cardiac defects 29
congenital dyserythropoietic anaemia 15
constipation 3
cordocentesis 58
corticosteroids 43, 58
co-trimoxazole 30, 55
craniospinal prophylaxis 23, 27
C reactive protein 18
creatinine 40
cryoprecipitate 63
cyclo-oxygenase activity 31
cyclophosphamide 34, 42, 49
cyclosporin A 53, 55
cystic fibrosis 55
cytogenic analysis 18, 21, 26, 34
cytogenic marker 20
cytomegalovirus 54, 56, 58
cytosine arabinoside 37
cytotoxic proteins 65, 69
cytotoxic therapy 5, 17, 19, 26–7, 30
  CHOP regime 49
  high dose 48, 50
  long term effects 50
  multiple myeloma 41
  myelodysplastic syndrome 37
  therapy-related myelodyplastic syndrome 34
  toxicity in acute leukaemia 28

dactylitis 11–12
danazol 33
deep vein thrombosis 45
deferiprone (L1) 13
dehydration 39, 61
dementia 59
desferrioxamine 13
desmopressin (DDAVP) 32–3, 44
dexamethasone 42, 62
diarrhoea 3, 54
diabetes mellitus 45
dialysis 41
direct sequence analysis 68
disseminated intravascular coagulation 31, 33,
  43–4, 58, 62–3
dissociative sensory loss 62
diuretics 17
Down's syndrome 24
doxorubicin 49, 50
drug resistance genes 69
dysfibrinogenaemia 43
dysphagia 2
dyspnoea 1, 25, 42

ecchymoses 20, 32
elderly people 58–9
encephalocele 6
endoscopy 8
enteropathy 6

gluten induced 6–7
enzymopathies 56
epistaxis 25, 32, 43–4
epithelial cell changes 7
Epstein-Barr virus 50
erythrocyte sedimentation 18, 40, 42, 59
erythroleukaemia 25
erythromelalgia 18
erythropoeisis 6
erythropoeitin 16, 37–8, 65
etoposide 37
exchange transfusion 58, 61
extramedullary haemopoeisis 19
extramedullary plasmacytoma 39

FAB (FrenchAmericanBritish) classification
  leukaemia 245
  myelodysplastic syndrome 36
FAB group 34, 36
facial redness 16–17
factor V Leiden mutation 45
familial macrocytosis 7
familial thrombophilia 45
Fanconi's anaemia 15, 24, 29
Fas ligand 68
fatigue 19, 20–1, 42, 47, 54
fava bean sensitivity 14
ferritin 1, 3, 13, 16, 18
fetoscopy 56
fever 31
fibrinogen 29
fludarabine 48
fluorescence activated cell sorter 69
folate deficiency 3, 5–9
folate metabolism 7
folates 6, 59
folic acid 6, 8–9, 13
  deficiency 59
fungal infection 28, 54

gall stones 11
Gaisbock's syndrome 18
gammaimmunoglobulin (IgG) 30, 39–40
gangrene 18
gastrectomy 8
gastric atrophy 59
gastric carcinoma 8
gastric polyps 8
gastritis 54
gastrointestinal bleeding 2, 32, 43–4, 59, 60
gene cloning 69
gene sequencing 69
gene therapy 55, 66, 67
  future of 65–6
gene transfer strategies 66
genetic counselling 57
genitourinary bleeding 32, 60
gingival bleeding 25
girdle syndrome 61
Glanzmann's thromboasthenia 30
globins 67
globin synthesis disorders 2
glossitis 1, 7, 59
glucose-6-phosphate dehydrogenase deficiency
  (G6PD) 14
gluten induced enteropathy 6–7
glycoprotein receptors 29
glycoproteins 29
gonadal dysfunction 7, 28
gout 16, 21
graft versus host disease 51–2, 54
gram negative septicaemia 63
granulocyte-colony stimulating factor 37–8, 52
growth retardation 13, 28
gum hypertrophy 25

H²-antagonists 6
haemanitic assays 2–3
haemarthrosis 43–4
haematological emergencies 60–4

haematology
  future of 65–7
haematuria 11, 44
haemoglobin 1, 10
  concentration 26
  elderly people 58
  neonatal 56
  recombinant 65, 67
haemoglobin electrophoresis 11
haemoglobinometers 65
haemoglobinopathies 10–14, 55, 57
haemolytic anaemia 9, 10–15
  neonatal 56
haemolytic uremic syndrome 31
haemophilia 32, 43–4, 55, 57
  future of treatment 68
  gene therapy 65
Haemophilus influenzae 11, 14
haemopoeisis 51
haemopoeitic growth factor 52, 69
haemopoeitic stem cells 67–8
haemopoeitic transplantation *see* bone marrow
  transplantation
haemorrhagic disease 58
haemorrhage 20–1, 40
haemosiderin 1, 6
haemostasis 29
  disorders 57
hair loss 28
hand and foot syndrome 11–12
haproglobins 6
hare lip 6
Hb Bart's hydrops fetalis syndrome 12–13
  see also thalassaemia
HB H disease 12–13, 57
  see also thalassaemia
Hb SC disease 11–12
  see also thalassaemia
headache 1, 16, 60
Heberden's nodes 3
Helicobacter pylori 48
heparin 31, 46, 63
heparinoids 33
hepatic sequestration crisis 11
hepatitis C 13
hepatosplenomegaly 13, 25, 42
hereditary anaemia 10–15, 67
hereditary spherocytosis 14
herpes virus 54–5, 63–4
heterodimeric transcription factor 69
hiatus hernia 3
HIV (human immunodeficiency virus) 30, 56,
  58
Hodgkin's disease 50, 52
homocysteine assay 8
HPA-1 antigen 58
human leucocyte antigen (HLA) 51, 52
  typing 21, 52, 55
human parvovirus B19 56, 61
hydrochloric acid 1
hydrops fetalis 56, 57
  see also thalassaemia
hydroxocobalamin 8
hydroxurea 7, 12, 17, 19, 21–2, 23, 37
hyperaesthesia 62
hypercalcaemia 39–41
hypercholesterolaemia 45
hypercoagulability 45
hyperfibrinogenaemia 45
hyperleucocytosis 60
hyperlipidaemia 45
hypermetabolism 19
hyper-reflexia 62
hypertension 17, 45
hypertonia 62
hyperuricaemia 26
hyperviscosity 39–40
  syndrome 42, 60–1
hypochromic anaemia 14, 12
hypofibrinogenaemia 43
hypoparathyroidism 5
hyposplenism 54, 55, 61, 64
hypothyroidism 5, 28, 54

hypotonia 62
hypoxaemia 17
hypoxia 61

idiopathic thrombocytopenic purpura 30
idiotypic vaccination 65
ileal resection 5, 8
immune dysfunction 54
immune paresis 39
immunisation 64
immunoglobulin 32–3, 39–40, 58, 64
immunophenotyping 26, 68
immunosuppresive therapy 51, 53, 55
infection 6, 10–11, 13, 27, 40–2, 47, 61
   anaemia 56–7
   atypical 54
   bacterial 34, 44, 54
   disseminated intravascular coagulation 63
   fungal 28, 54
   impaired immunity 63–4
   viral 30, 54–5, 58
   Yersinia spp. 13
infectious mononucleosis 30
infertility 28, 54
interferon alfa 19, 21–2, 41, 65
interleukin 6 39
intermittent claudication 59
intestinal stagnant loop syndrome 5
intracerebral bleeding 46
intracranial bleeding 32, 58
intrauterine fetal death 63
intrauterine transfusion 56, 58
intravascular transfusion 56
intrinsic factor 5
   antibodies 8
iron
   accumulation 13
   daily requirements 1
   deficiency 1–4, 58–9
   metabolism 1
   overload 19
   replacement therapy 34
   serum 59
iron chelation therapy 37
iron sorbitol 4
irradiation 20, 24, 27

jaundice 6, 14, 54
   see also kernicterus

karyotypic evolution 34
kernicterus 56
Kleinfelter's syndrome 24
Kelihauer test 56
koilonychia 1, 59

lactation 1
lactic dehydrogenase 6, 21, 49
laser treatment 12
legionella 54
leg ulcers 11, 13, 61
lethargy 1, 40, 59
leucocytosis 36
leucoerythroblastosis 19
leucopenia 56
leucostasis 21
leukaemia 43
   acute 24–8, 52
   acute promyelocytic 63, 69
   chronic lymphocytic 39, 42, 47–8, 63
   chronic myeloid 20–3, 52, 69
   chronic myelomonocytic 35, 37
   erythroleukaemia 25
   FAB classification 24–5
   future of treatment 68–9
   megakaryoblastic 25
   plasma cell 39, 42
Leukaemia Research Fund 21
leukaemic skin deposits 25, 37

leukaemic transformation
   myelodysplastic syndrome 36
ligands 66, 68
liver biopsy 13
liver damage 13, 62
liver disease 3, 5, 43–4
liver transplantation 68
lumbar puncture 26
lung cancer 52
lung syndrome 1112
lupus anticoagulants 45
lymphadenopathy 21, 25–6, 42, 47–8, 50
lymphocytes 39, 42, 47
lymphocytic leukaemia
   acute 24–8, 52
   chronic 39, 42, 47–8, 63
lymphoma 42
   AIDS-related 50
   Ann Arbor staging 47
   Burkitt's 49
   diffuse large cell 49
   follicular 47–8
   gene therapy 65
   Hodgkin's 50
   lymphoblastic 49
   malignant 39, 47–50
   non-Hodgkin's 42, 47–50
lymphopenia 56
lymphoplasmocytoid bone marrow infiltration 42
lymphoproliferative disorders 39–42, 44
   heavy chain disease 42
lytic bone lesions 26, 39–40, 62

macrocytic anaemia 59, 34, 59
macrocytosis 59, 34
   familial 7
magnetic resonance imaging 62
malabsorption 2–3, 6, 54, 59
malaria 57
malignancy 59
malignant lymphoma *see* lymphomas
maltomas (mucosal associated lymphoid tumours) 48
mammalian cell culture 68, 69
May-Heggelin anomaly 29–30
mediastinal mass 25–6, 49
Medical Research Council trials 21, 27
megakaryoblastic leukaemia 25
megakaryocytes 29, 34
megaloblastic anaemia 6, 59
melphalan 41–2
meningeal syndrome 25
meningococcal septicaemia 44
menorrhagia 25, 32, 43
menstruation 1–2
mental retardation 13
metabolic disorders 52
methotrexate 5, 23, 27, 53
methylprednisolone 42
microcytic anaemia 14
microvascular haemolysis 31
microvascular occlusion 18
molecular biology 65–9
molecular studies 26
monoclonal antibodies 48, 53, 68
monoclonal gammopathy 39–41
monoclonal immunoglobulin 39, 60
monocytosis 34
M proteins 39–41
mucocutaneous bleeding 32, 43
mucosal ulceration 54
mucositis 28, 54
multiple myeloma 39–42, 52
   management 40
   plateau phase 40–1
   smouldering 39–40
mycoplasma 54
myelodysplasia 5, 7–8, 18, 52
myelodysplastic syndrome 34–8, 44, 59
   FAB classification 36
   international prognostic scoring system 37

management 37–8
myelofibrosis 17–18, 23
   idiopathic 19
myeloma 8, 60
myeloproliferative disorders 18, 36, 44–5
myelosuppression 28, 53, 54
myocardial damage 13
myocardial infarction 7, 45
myxoedema 5

National Blood Transfusion Service 52
nausea 3, 28, 54
Neisseria meningitidis 11, 14
neonatal alloimmune thrombocytopenia 58
neonatal anaemia 56
neonatal haemorrhagic disease 58
neonatal jaundice 14
neonatal period 5, 7
neonatal thrombocytopenia 29, 31, 58
neural tube defects 6–8
neurological disease 11–12, 42
neuropathy 6, 28, 40
neutropenia 13, 25–6, 34, 40
   severe 27
night sweats 47
nitrous oxide anaesthesia 5
non-Hodgkin's lymphomas 47–50, 52
   AIDS-related 50
   extranodal (maltoma) 48
   gene therapy 65
   high grade 49
   intermediate grade 49
   nodal 47–8
non-steroidal analgesia 3, 31, 43, 59
normochromic normocytic anaemia 40, 56, 59
nose bleeds *see* epistaxis
nucleic acid sequence analysis 67
nystagmus 60

obesity 17
occlusive vascular lesions 16
occult blood 3
oesophageal varices 19
oesophageal web 2, 59
oesophagitis 54
opiates 41, 61
oral contraceptives 45
organ infiltration 25
osteoarthritis 3
osteoclasis 39
osteoblastosis 39
osteogenesis imperfecta 24
osteolytic lesions 39–40
osteomyelitis 10
osteoporosis 40

p210 protein 21
packed cell volume 16–17
pallor 6, 25, 59
pancreatic damage 13
pancytopenia 67, 23. 26
paraproteinaemia 5, 7
paraproteins 39–42
parietal cell antibodies 8
parvovirus B19 56, 61
pathological fractures 39
penicillamine 30
penicillin 11, 14, 55
   prophylaxis 64
pentamidine 55
peripheral blood stem cell transplantation 51–2
peripheral neuropathy 6
peripheral oedema 59
peripheral vascular disease 45
pernicious anaemia 5–7, 8, 59
petechiae 62
pharyngeal web 2
Philadelphia chromosome 20, 26
phospholipids 45
placental abruption 63

Index

plasma
  exchange 32
  fresh frozen 26, 32, 46, 63
  viscosity 40
plasma cell dyscrasias 39–42
plasma cell leukaemia 39, 42
plasma cells 42
plasmacytoid lymphocytes 42
plasmacytoma 39, 42
plasmapheresis 42, 61
plasma proteins 60
plasmids 65, 67
platelet concentrate 26
platelet count 18, 21, 26, 43
platelet derived growth factor 29
platelet disorders 29–33, 43–4
  acquired 29–30
  congenital 30–1
  management 32–3
platelet factor 4 31
platelet transfusions 32, 37, 58, 63
pneumococcal sepsis 55, 57
Pneumocystis carinii 55
pneumocystis pneumonia 54
pneumonitis 54
polycythaemia 16–18, 60
polymerase chain reaction 65–9
portal hypertension 19
positive pressure isolation 54
post-transfusion purpura 31, 33
postviral thrombocytopenia 32
prednisolone 32–3, 41, 42, 49, 54
pre-eclampsia 63
pregnancy
  anticoagulation therapy 46
  iron deficiency anaemia 12
  chronic myeloid leukaemia 21
  macrocytosis 5, 7
  prenatal screening 57, 67–8
  preventing folate deficiency 8
  sickle cell disease 11
  thalassaemia 13
  venous thrombosis 45
  vitamin B12 deficiency 6
prenatal diagnosis 67–8
prenatal treatment 68
  see also intrauterine transfusion
priapism 11, 21, 61
procoagulants 62
prostatic specific antigen 62
protein C 45–6
protein electrophoresis 62
protein engineering 69
protein S 456
proteinuria 40
prothrombin time 43, 46, 63
protoporphyrin 67
pruritus 16, 50
psychiatric abnormality 6
psychological disturbance 54
pulmonary angiography 45
pulmonary disease 11–12
pulmonary embolism 45
purpura 21, 30–3, 40
pyruvate kinase deficiency 14

QALY (quality of life adjusted years) analysis
  55

radiation exposure 20, 24, 34
radioactive vitamin B12 absorption studies 8
radioactive phosphorus 17
radiotherapy
  Hodgkin's disease 50
  maltomas 48
  multiple myeloma 41
  myelofibrosis 19
  plasmocytoma 42
rash 54
reactive thrombocytosis 18–19
recombinant blood products 69

recombinant coagulation factor VII 68
recombinant growth factors 37
recombinant haemoglobin 65, 67
recombinant human factor VIII 68
recombinant proteins 69
red cell
  aplasia 5, 7
  enzyme defects 14
  folate 7, 59
  fragmentation 31
  mass 16
  membrane defects 14–15
  metabolic pathways 14
  rouleaux 40
  (packed) transfusion 27, 37
Reed Sternberg cell 47
refractory anaemia 36
rehydration 41
rejection 51–2
renal disease 43–4
renal failure 11–12, 39, 49, 62
renal impairment 26, 31, 40, 61
renal lesions 17
reticulocytosis 5, 31
retinal bleeding 32, 42
retinal damage 11, 13, 21, 61
retinoic acid analogues 37
retinoic acid receptor gene 69
retroviral vectors 66
rhesus incompatibility 56
rheumatoid disease 3
ricin 48
root compression 62
rubella 56, 58
Russell's viper venom test 45

secondary malignancy 28, 59, 62
sequestration episodes 11, 61
sicca syndrome 54
sickle cell disease 52, 57, 67
  anaemia 9, 10–12
  β thalassaemia 10–11, 57
  crises 11–12, 57, 61
  gene 10
  gene therapy 65
sickling disorders 10–12
sideroblastic anaemia 2–3
Sögren's syndrome 48
skeletal changes 13
skeletal survey 40
skin atrophy 1, 54
skin staining 4
smoking 17, 45
spina bifida 6
spinal cord compression 40, 62
splenectomy
  chronic myeloid leukaemia 23
  hereditary spherocytosis 14
  Hodgkin's disease 50
  myelofibrosis 19
  sickle cell disease 12
  thalassaemia 14
  thrombocythaemia 18
  thrombocytopenia 32
splenic sequestration crisis 11, 57, 61
splenomegaly
  acquired bleeding disorders 44
  chronic myeloid leukaemia 20–1, 23
  myelodysplastic syndrome 34, 36
  myelofibrosis 19
  polycythaemia 16
  thalassaemia 12–14
  thrombocythaemia 18
  thrombocytopenia 31
stem cell rescue 48, 50
stem cell surgery 67–8
stem cell transplantation *see* bone marrow
    transplantation
steroids 43–4, 48, 54
stillbirth 57
stomatitis 1, 59
Streptococcus pneumoniae 11, 14

stress erythrocytosis 18
stroke 45
subconjunctival bleeding 32
surgery 45
syphilis 56
systemic lupus erythematosus 30
sweating 20–1, 23
  night 47

tachycardia 2
target cells 65–6
TAR syndrome 29
taste disturbance 1
testicular cancer 52
testicular enlargement 25
thalassaemia 2–3, 10–14, 52, 57, 67
  distribution 12
  features 57
  inheritance 12
  intermedia 13
thrombin time 43
thrombocythaemia 18–19
thrombocytopenia 23, 25–6, 34, 40, 43–4
  HIV 56
  maternal autoimmune 58
  neonatal 58
  postviral 32
thrombocytopenia-absent radii (TAR)
    syndrome 29
thrombocytosis 20, 31
thromboembolism 45
thromboplastin time 45
thrombopoeitin 29, 65, 69
thromboprophylaxis 45
thrombosis 45
thrombotic thrombocytopenia purpura 31
thrombophlebitis 45
thyroid deficiency 7
  see also hypothyroidism, myxoedema
tinnitus 1
tissue infection 10–11
tissue ischaemia 62
toxoplasmosis 54, 56, 58
tranexamic acid 32–3
transcobalamin 11 deficiency 5
transferrin 1, 59
tuberculosis, abdominal 6

umbilical cord blood 55
uraemia 31
urea 40
urine electrophoresis 40

vascular occlusion 11, 18–19, 61
vector systems 65–6
veganism 5, 8
venesection 17
venogram 45
venous congestion 42
veno-occlusive disease 54
venous thrombosis 7, 45, 62
ventilation perfusion scanning 45
vertebral disc calcification 13
vertigo 60
vinca alkaloids 33
  vincristine 42, 49
viral infection 30
viruses 24
  cytomegalovirus 54, 56
  Epstein-Barr 50
  herpes 54–5
  HIV 30, 56
  human parvovirus B19 56, 61
  recombinant 65
visual disturbance 6, 21, 40, 42, 60
vitamin B12 5–7, 8, 59
vitiligo 5–6
vitamin C 13, 44
vitamin D3 analogues 37
vitamin K 44, 46

deficiency 58
vomiting 28, 54

warfarin 33, 43, 46, 58
  international normalised ratio 46

Waldenström's macroglobulinaemia 39, 42, 60
weight loss 19, 20–1, 42, 47
white cell count 26
von Willebrand's disease 30, 32, 43
von Willebrand's factor 29, 31
Wiskott-Aldrich's syndrome 21, 30

X gal staining 66
X-linked disorder 30

Yersinia spp. infection 13

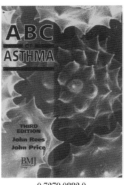
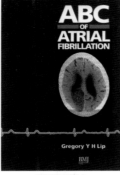
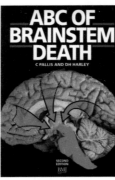
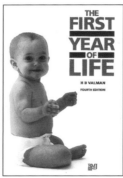
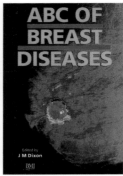
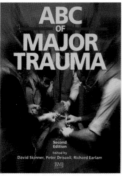
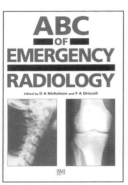
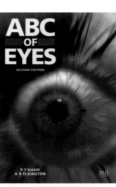
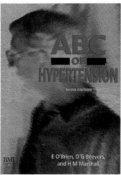
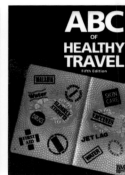
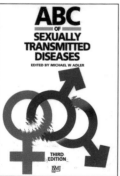
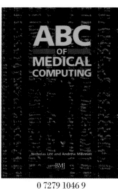
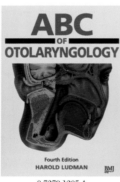
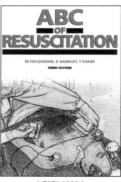
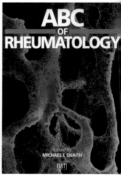
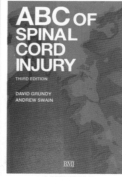
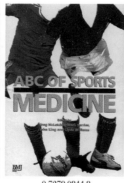
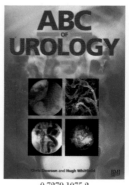
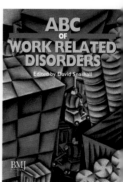
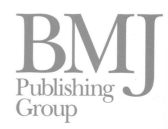